CLINICAL PRECISION PRACTICES OF MODERN MEDICINE

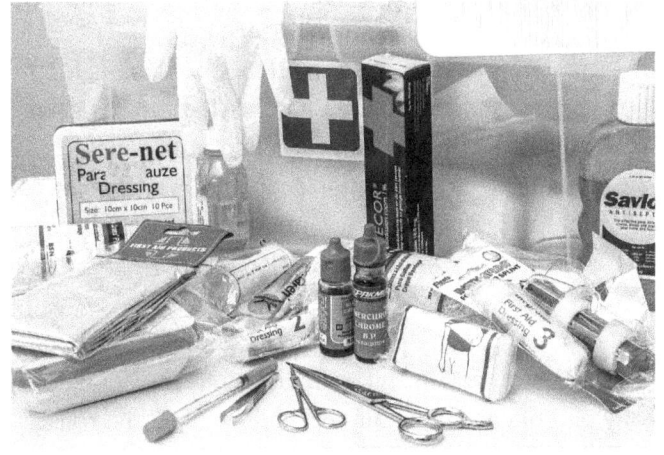

Ultimate Guide On How To Administer Safe IV and Im Injection

TABLE OF CONTENTS

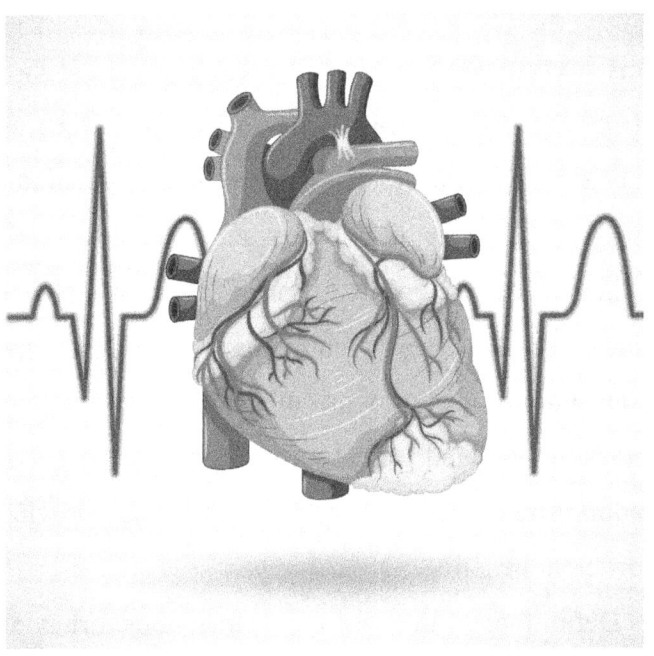

CHAPTER 1:

INTRODUCTION

1.1 Overview Of Intravenous (Iv) And Intramuscular (Im) Injections: As far as healthcare is concerned, there are several important ways through which drugs and fluids can be administered to the body; one such way includes intravascular and intramuscular injections. Depending on the type of medicine, speed of transmission, and patient's condition these routes of administration can be preferred since they provide different benefits.

- Definition: In the case of IV injections, drugs or fluids are introduced directly into the bloodstream through a vein.

- Speed of Action: Fast acting and thus suitable for emergency use or medications that need rapid systemic effects.

- Common Uses: Fluids administration, chemotherapy, antibiotics, and any drugs that need careful dose delivery.

Intramuscular (IM) Injections:
- Definition: Injecting a medication intramuscularly involves placing it in the muscles underneath the skin.
- Absorption Rate: Compared to IV, generally slower absorption results in a more sustained release of drug from the gut.
- Common Uses: Vaccine administration, specific antibiotics, prolonged-release medication, as well as some hormone therapy drugs.

Key Considerations:
The aseptic technique is extremely critical for IV injection because it bypasses the blood stream thereby reducing the the chances of infections.

- IM injections require needles of adequate length, proper sites of injection, and consideration for the patient's comfort so that drugs are absorbed well enough.

- These two routes required an depth understanding of anatomy, drug compatibility, and patient factors to prevent complications that might arise out of ignorance.

Challenges:

- If not administered carefully, intravenous injections can cause infection, thrombosis, and infiltration.

- Therefore, IM injection is precise avoiding injuries on nerves or vessels with consideration of a patient's aspects, for example, his/her age; as well as his/her muscles.

1. 2 Importance Of Safe Administration

Health care delivery depends in a variety of ways on the safe administration of IV and IM injections that affects patients' outcome at a large scale, set health care standards as well and determine the quality of health care practice. Concisely, significance may be explained as:

1. Patient Safety and Well-being:
- Prevents the occurrence of allergenic reactions, communicable diseases such as HIV, AIDS, and hepatitis, and other risks associated with anesthetic procedures.
- Ensure better safety during drug administration and improve safety in healthcare settings.

2. Optimal Medication Delivery:
- It provides appropriate medication for particular parts of the body at maximal absorption points.
- It boosts the efficacy of drugs in enhancing appropriate treatment results.

3. Prevention Of Infections:

- Bloodstream infections are very common issues in this setting during IV administration and aseptic technique compliance plays a major role in their prevention.

- Improvement of patient's health and reducing cases of local infections in Intramuscular (IM) injections require proper hygiene.

4. Complication Minimization:

- Safe administration practice such as avoidance of complication like tissue irritations and extravasation infiltration assists in minimizing complication.

- Avoiding systemic complications that may take the drugs of course.

5. Therapeutic Efficiency:

- It enhances efficiency in the treatment plan, facilitating the achievement of the therapeutic goals within the schedule.

- Enhances predictability and reliability of drugs, streamlines provision of patient care.

6. Adherence To Standards And Regulations:

- Considers health care laws and sets out a rule that the provider has to follow.

- Ensures that there are no liability issues arising from the wrong dosage errors while injecting.

7. Professional Integrity And Trust:

- It encourages caregivers to preserve standards of integrity, and this will instill faith among patients and other participants in the same venture.

- Builds loyalty with practitioners and their clients.

8. Patient Education And Empowerment:

- Educates the patients on how they should help themselves in treating the disease, and gives them the confidence to work together and take medicines that have been prescribed.

- It is important that patients are educated on injection procedures and possible complications to improve their understanding of their healthcare process.

9. Efficient Emergency Response:

- Ensures smooth emergency response when unexpected reactions or complications occur during injection administration.

- Readiness coupled with observance of security rules enhances quick responses or remedies.

10. Continuous Quality Improvement:

- Encourages the quality improvement process that is continuous within healthcare by making sure that the knowledge base among healthcare professionals is continuously updated.

- Improves injection practices, enhancing patient care.

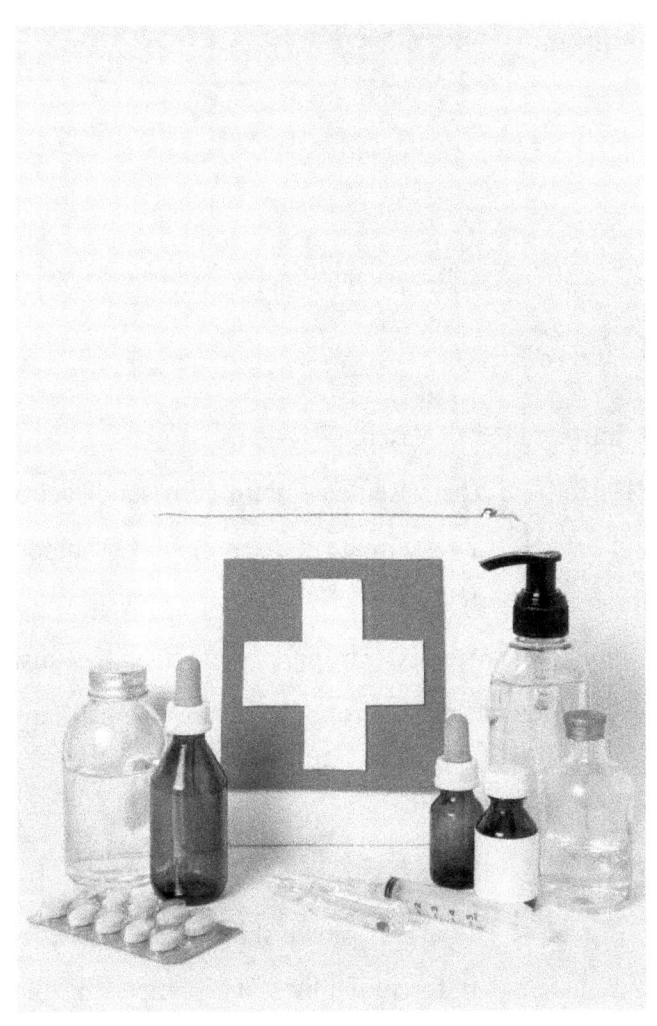

CHAPTER 2: ANATOMY AND PHYSIOLOGY

2.1 Understanding Veins and Arteries

1. Introduction to Vascular System:

- Definition: The vascular system consists of veins and arteries that facilitate the circulation of blood around the body.

- Function: Arteries transport blood that has just been oxygenated far from the heart, while veins send back de-oxygenated blood.

2. Arteries:

- Structure: The arteries have thick muscular walls to hold all that forceful blood out-pumped by the heart.

- Function: Distributes oxygenated blood through the body except in the pulmonary arteries.

- Elasticity: Elastic arteries are flexible and expandable so they stretch as required by the varying fluid pressures associated with different blood flows.

3. Types Of Arteries:
- Elastic Arteries: Vessels around the heart (such as the aorta), which dilate and recoil to keep blood flowing at an even rate.
- Muscular Arteries: Have thicker muscles that assist in the regulation of the blood flow towards the body's particular organs.

4. Veins:
- Structure: Unlike the arterial system, veins have thin walls and large lumen and therefore, they work under lower pressure.
- Function: This blood is deoxygenated, except for the pulmonary veins which transport oxygen-rich blood back to the heart.
- Valves: One-way valves are found in most veins to ensure there is no reversal flow of blood.

5. Types Of Veins:

- Superficial Veins: Usually close to the body surface, sometimes seen through the skin.

- Deep Veins: Parallel to arteries and carrying of the bulk of blood volume.

6. Blood Circulation:

- Systemic Circulation: The heart takes in oxygenified blood through arteries and gives deoxygenated blood to the heart through veins.

- Pulmonary Circulation: The first set of vessels is called pulmonary arteries that carry deoxygenated blood to the lungs while pulmonary veins bring back oxygenated blood to the heart.

7. Capillaries:

- Connection: Capillaries link arteries to veins, which is where transfer of nutrients, oxygen, and waste occurs between tissues. blood system; veins; arteries

- Microcirculation: Microcirculation of tissues is provided by a dense capillary net.

8. Factors Influencing Blood Flow:
- Blood Pressure: Blood is forced through the body's system by arterial pressure.
- Vein Function: Valves are used while veins depend on valves as well as the contraction of skeletal muscles in enabling blood to flow back to the heart.

9. Clinical Significance:
- Blood Draws and IV Access: This is because veins are usually preferred because they can easily be accessed.
- Arterial Diseases: Blood clips or arterial diseases like atherosclerosis in most cases lead to cardiovascular problems by impairing or interfering with proper blood circulation.

10. Maintenance Of Cardiovascular Health:

- Lifestyle Factors: A healthy diet, exercise, and not smoking help keep the vessels and blood vessels in good condition.

- Medical Interventions: Vascular problems can be controlled using medications or surgical intervention, to prevent heart disease as well.

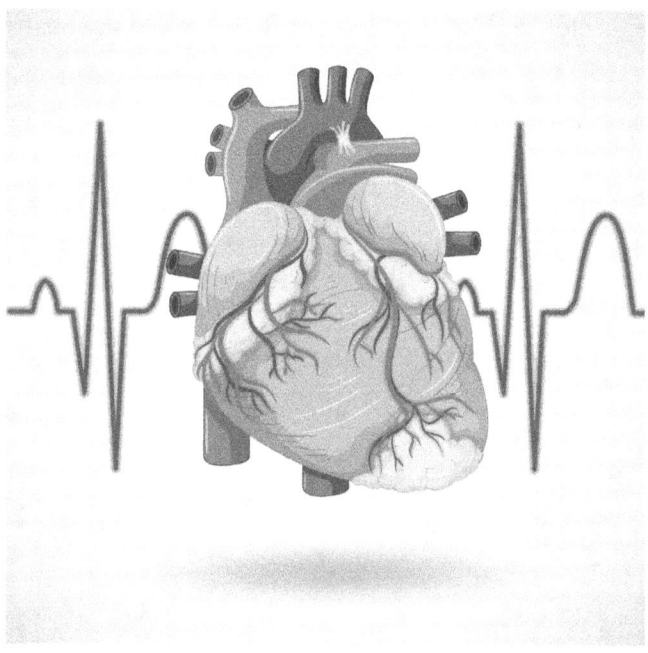

2.2 Anatomy Of The Muscles For Im Injection.

1. Introduction to Intramuscular (IM) Injections:

- Definition: This is basically when someone injects some form of medicine directly into the muscles beneath their skin through a needle.

- Purpose: Used frequently for drugs of controlled release or when any irritant tissue is involved with subcutaneous applications.

2. Target Muscles For Im Injections:

- Deltoid Muscle: Deltoid which is located in the arm above is often used for a small amount of medication.

- Ventrogluteal Muscle: Preferably, such deep IM injections are administered in the area around the hip as the muscle at this site is thick.

- Vastus Lateralis: It is located in a thigh and is often applied for pediatric or extensive cases.

3. Anatomy Of The Muscles:

- Deltoid Muscle: Around the shoulder joint, multiple muscles meet up to form the round shape.
- Ventrogluteal Muscle: This is made of two muscles – gluteus medius and minimus, giving it a thick and vascular tissue that allows for needle puncture.
- Vastus Lateralis: It is located at the side or lateral part of the thigh, offering a convenient and secure injection spot.

4. Preparing For Im Injections:

- Identifying Landmarks: Locate the injection site by palpating bony landmarks and muscle borders.
- Patient Positioning: Positioning the patient in such a way relaxes the muscles making easy syringe injections possible.

5. Deltoid Muscle:

- Landmarks: The injection should be in the middle third of the muscle, under the acromion process.

- Volume Limit: Lower volume (generally no more than 2 mL), to prevent pressure-related issues.

6. Ventrogluteal Muscle:
- Landmarks: Accurate site selection requires proper identification of the greater trochanter, anterior superior iliac spine, and iliac crest.
- Advantages: Deep location diminishes the chances of puncturing blood vessels and veins.

7. Vastus Lateralis:
- Landmarks: Inject half of them in the middle third of the thigh.
- Use in Pediatrics: This is because of the great muscle mass available in pediatric patients most of the time.

8. Needle Insertion Technique:
- Insertion Angle: Generally at ninety degrees for adults, but it depends on patient factors and body mass.

- Z-Track Method: A way to reduce drug diffusion into the subcutaneous tissues, which is often used during ventrolateral injections.

9. Considerations For IM Injections:

- Needle Length: Use it by taking into consideration the level of body fat thickness of adipose tissues while adjusting for muscle mass.
- Aspiration: To avoid administration of blood through the vein, ensure there are no drops of blood when you are about to inject.

10. Potential Complications:

- Pain and Discomfort: Provision of patient education and appropriate strategy to minimize pain.
- Infection Risk: Following the aseptic technique prevents infections at the injection site.

HEART ANATOMY

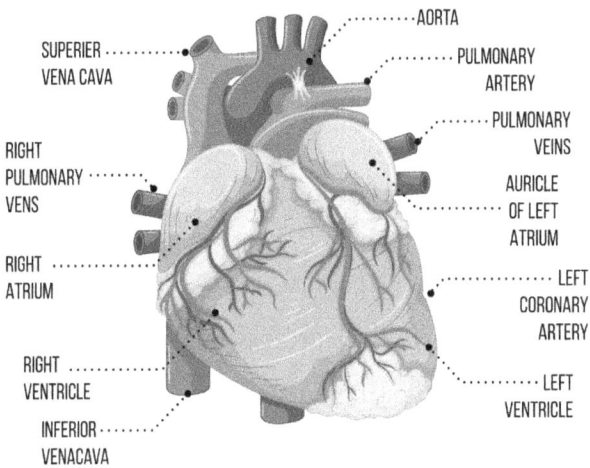

SUPERIER
VENA CAVA

AORTA

PULMONARY
ARTERY

PULMONARY
VEINS

RIGHT
PULMONARY
VENS

AURICLE
OF LEFT
ATRIUM

RIGHT
ATRIUM

LEFT
CORONARY
ARTERY

RIGHT
VENTRICLE

LEFT
VENTRICLE

INFERIOR
VENACAVA

CHAPTER 3: INJECTION EQUIPMENT AND SUPPLIES

3.1 Needles: Types and Sizes

1. Introduction to Needles:

- Definition: Medical professionals use needles as small pointed instruments serving many functions such as injection and retrieval of blood samples.

- Components: Comprises a hub, a shaft, and a beveled head.

2. Needle Gauge:

- Definition: Gauge is the diameter of the needle shaft.

- Inverse Relationship: In general, the smaller the gauge number, the larger the diameter; in reverse order.

- Common Gauges: Some of the common sizes are 18G (bigger) and 30G (smaller).

3. Needle Length:

- Definition: This is the measurement of length, i.e., the distance between the point on the tip and the bottom of its axis.

- Varied Lengths: From very short, for example, 3/8 inch to longer lengths such as 3 inches.

- Selection Criteria: Based on the injection site, patient factors, and procedure.

4. Types Of Needles:

A. Hypodermic Needles:

- General Use: Used frequently for injection and venipuncture.

- Beveled Tip: Helps easy piercing into the skin.

B. Insulin Needles:

- Specialized: Designed specifically for insulin administration.

- Short Length: Smaller, usually shorter than eight millimeters.

C. Intramuscular (IM) Needles:

- Length: Needles longer than this (such as an inch or so), for example, needed to be used so that they can get through the layer of fat to the deepest layers of the underlying muscle tissue.

- Gauge: For instance, 20g up to 25g is often used with the thinner ones.

D. Subcutaneous (SubQ) Needles:

- Length: Smaller-sized needles (e.g., between 3/- and 1 inch) for intracellular injections into the fatty tissue below-skin

- Gauge: Smaller gauge, say 25G to 30G.

E. Spinal Needles:

- Specialized: For spinal and epidural processes.

- Beveled Tip: It allows accurate insertion into the spinal canal.

F. Butterfly Needles (Winged Infusion Sets):

- Design: Flexible tubing with handles.

- Use: Inserted into the fragile veins or for continuous blood drawing.

G. Huber Needles:
- Design: They are tailored and made for use with implantable venous ports.
- Angled Tip: Enables the best entrance to the port without damaging the septum.

5. Selection Considerations:
- Patient Factors: Be mindful of the age, size, and preferences of the patient.
- Medication Characteristics: Larger gauge needles can help to administer thicker or viscous medications.
- Injection Site: It is important to have different needle types and sizes depending on the site such as muscle, subcutaneous, or intravenous.

6. Safety Features:
- Needle Safety Devices: The design of various mechanisms (for instance, retractable needles)

aimed at limiting the likelihood of needlestick injuries.

- Preventing Accidental Exposure: Safety features can promote the safety of healthcare workers.

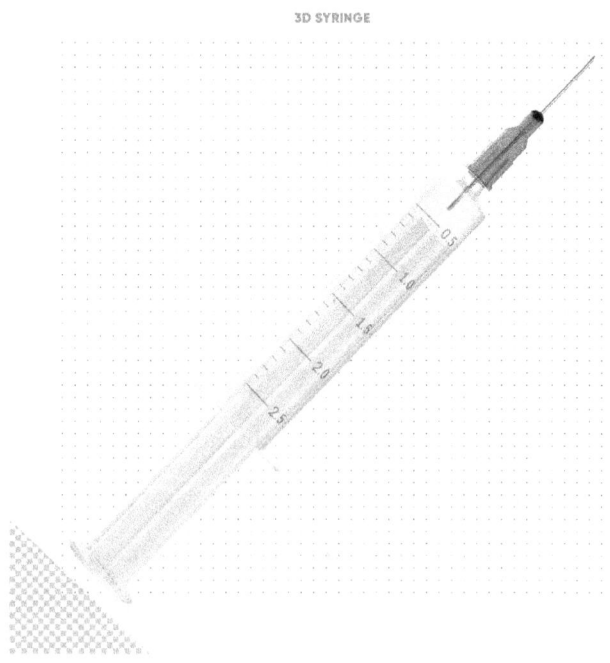

3D SYRINGE

3.2 Syringes: Selection And Use

1. Introduction to Syringes:
- Definition: Syringes are instruments that withdraw, quantify, and inject fluids and drugs.
- Components: Barrel with a plunger and needle tip.

2. Syringe Sizes:
- Volume Capacity: Different volumes starting from 0.5 ml up to 60 ml and above.
- Selection Criteria: According to the amount of medication to be applied.

3. Types of Syringes:
A. Standard Disposable Syringes:
- Single Use: Single-use ones intended for preventing contamination.
- Common Sizes: For different purposes, range from 1 mL – 10 mL.

B. Insulin Syringes:
- Specific Design: Smaller volume calibrated versions for insulin dosing.

- Unit Markings: Specially marked in Insulin units for accurate measurement.

C. Tuberculin Syringes:
- Calibration: These are graduated in tenths of a milliliter for measuring small volumes accurately.
- Common Use: Administer small medication doses including tuberculin skin tests.

D. Prefilled Syringes:
- Preloaded Medication: Comes in pre-loaded dosages of one specific medicine.
- Reduced Risk of Contamination: Reduces the chances of dosage errors and contaminations.

4. Syringe Components:
A. Barrel:
- Volume Graduations: Measured by marked in milliliters or cubic centimeters for accurate measurement.
- Material: They are made out of plastic or glass which is transparent to allow viewing inside readily.

B. Plunger:

- Operation: A device used to either ingress or egress fluids into/from the barrel.

- Rubber or Silicone Seal: Gives accurate reading to ensure a tight seal when measuring for dose-accurate.

C. Tip:

- Luer Lock or Slip: Various forms of locking needles to the syringe.

- Compatibility: Compatible with a variety of needle kinds.

5. Syringe Use:

A. Medication Draw-up:

- Aspiration Technique: Avoiding contamination when drawing medication in a syringe.

- Air Removal: Evacuate the air bubbles for correct determination of dosage.

B. Needle Attachment:

- Secure Attachment: Fasten the needle on the syringe by ensuring it is firmly in place.
- Luer Lock vs. Slip Tip: Type based on the needle and procedure selection.

C. Administration Techniques:

- Intramuscular (IM), Subcutaneous (SubQ), Intradermal (ID), Intravenous (IV): Multiple approaches depending upon the location of injection.
- Angle of Insertion: Angle adjustment is dependent upon the injection site and procedure.

6. Safety Considerations:

- Single-Use Policy: Using single-use syringes as per the principle of avoiding cross infection.
- Needle Safety Features: Employing syringe safety devices to minimize needlestick injury rates.

7. Waste Disposal:

- Sharps Container: Safe disposal of used syringes, and use of sharps for safe handling purposes.

- Adherence to Protocols: Safely follow the prescribed standards of institutions and regulators for waste disposal.

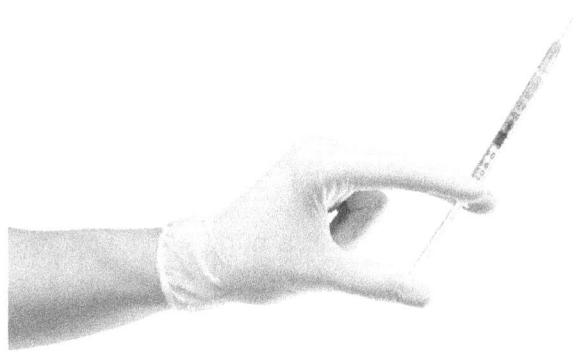

3.3 Additional (Alcohol Swaps, Gauze, Etc)

1. Alcohol Swabs:
- Purpose: Disinfect the injection site before injecting.
- Antiseptic Properties: They contain isopropyl alcohol to prevent infections.
- Technique: Using gauze or towel wipes, clean the skin in circular motions moving from inside out for optimum disinfection.
- Disposable: Unique disposable containers for contamination prevention.

2. Gauze Pads:
- Purpose: Used for different purposes in and after performing injection.
- Cleaning: Used as post-alcohol swab cleaning at the injection's spot."
- Pressure Application: It is applied on the injection site afterward, to reduce bleeding and bruise.
- Absorbent: Absorbs extra blood and fluid.

3. Bandages Or Adhesive Strips:

- Purpose: Covered on the injection site to prevent contamination with soil and bacteria.

- Pressure Application: It assists in preserving the injection area pressure.

- Comfort: The caregiver is there to offer support and shield the patient after the injection has been done.

4. Sterile Gloves:

- Purpose: As an item worn by healthcare providers to ensure asepsis.

- Protection: It stops microorganisms from being transferred from the healthcare giver into the beneficiary and also from the beneficiary into the healthcare as well.

- Disposable: One-time use gloves to guarantee sterility.

5. Sharps Container:

- Purpose: A separate container that ensures proper disposal of used needles, syringes, and sharp instruments.

- Safety: It reduces the probability of needlestick injuries and helps keep used and toxic items away from people.

- Compliance: Safety procedures to be followed in disposing of needles or sharps.

6. Tourniquet:

- Purpose: It is used to mark the veins visible so that they can be punctured easily.

- Application: Located close to the intended injection or blood sampling points with a temporary effect on blood flow.

- Caution: Be applied for short intervals so that circulation is maintained.

7. Biohazard Bag:

- Purpose: Getting rid of contamination in a safe manner.

- Color Coding: These are usually identified by the biohazard sign and color coding which can denote a biohazard.
- Segregation: Properly disposes of biohazardous waste.

8. Adhesive Bandages (Plasters):
- Purpose: Put over the injection site to avoid infection and to ease pain.
- Variety: Different sizes are available for use on various injection sites.
- Patient Comfort: Enhances patient comfort post-injection.

9. Transparent Film Dressing:
- Purpose: In this case, they act as a sterile cover over the injection site.
- Visibility: Due to their semi-transparent nature, healthcare providers can easily evaluate the injection site by looking through the dressing.
- Barrier Protection: It acts as a protection from contaminants but makes the object visible.

10. Marker Pen:
- Purpose: To specify injection sites and identify skin locations for assessments.
- Precision: The fine-pointed marker enables precise markings.
- Temporary Markings: Therefore, marks must be easily temporary and easy to remove.

CHAPTER 4: INFECTION CONTROL

4. 1. Hand Hygiene And Gloves Use.

1. Hand Hygiene:

- Importance: Crucial in stopping infection transmission at a hospital.

- Methods:

- Handwashing:

- Duration: A minimum of 20 seconds using soap and water.

- Steps: Cover all areas of fingertips, wrists, and fingernails.

- Hand Sanitization:

- Alcohol-Based: Effective disinfection – contains at least 60% alcohol.

- Application: Massage vigorously into moist hands and leave to dry.

2. When to Perform Hand Hygiene:

- Before Patient Contact:

- Any physical contact with a patient prior.

- before putting on gloves for a particular procedure.

- After Patient Contact:

- Following the treatment of any patient or physical contact with them.

- After removing gloves.

- Other Instances:

- After using the restroom.

- Before and after eating.

- When touching contaminated surfaces or objects after that.

3. Glove Use:

- Purpose: Prevents health care providers or patients against contamination.

- Selection Criteria:

- Material: Select the best-fitting gloves depending on the methodology used.

- Size: Have a tight fit, but while preserving flexibility.

- When to Wear Gloves:

- Direct Patient Contact:

- For instance, body fluid leakages, wound exposure, and even contact with blood during the procedures.

- Upon contact with mucous membranes or non-intact skin.

- Environmental Contact:

- Handling contaminated surfaces or objects.

- Cleaning and disinfection activities.

4. Proper Glove Application:

- Washing Hands: Use hand hygiene before putting on gloves,

- Selecting Gloves: Select among the types as well as select the most fitting size for the glove.

- Donning Sequence: Take precautions while putting on the gloves do not contaminate the outwear.

5. During Glove Use:

- Avoid Touching Face: Gloves should not be allowed to touch the face, hair, and surfaces while using them.

- Proper Technique: Change gloves after every task or patient contact.

- Limitation: Hand washing is still a necessity even with gloves.

6. Glove Removal:

- Sequence:

- Grip and Peel: Pull back and take hold of one half-glove with your fingers near the wrist; turn this side inside out.

- Hold in Gloved Hand: Put the removed glove into one of the gloves.

- Un-gloved Hand: Lift other gloves and turn them outwards.

- Dispose: Do not throw away gloves anywhere except in a proper trash bin.

7. Hand Hygiene After Glove Removal:

- Importance: For instance, as a way of reducing the risk of any contamination due to glove removal.

- Use of Hand Sanitizer: Use alcohol-based hand sanitizers if soap and water are unavailable.

8. Compliance with Protocols:

- Institutional Policies: Compliance with hand hygiene and glove use policies of health care facility.

- Regulatory Guidelines: Stick to established norms set forth by public health offices.

9. Educating Healthcare Providers:

- Training: Offer continuous education about good hand hygiene and glove usage.

- Awareness: The need for following preventive measures to prevent infection should be stressed.

4.2 Sterile Technique

1. Definition:

- Purpose: The set of activities meant to keep an infection-free atmosphere and to prevent the entry of micro-organisms in certain places which may cause infections.

- Applications: For use in medical procedures including those for surgery, wound care, etc.

2. Key Principles:

A. Hand Hygiene:

- Thorough Washing: Sterile activities should be performed after washing the hands with soap and water or the use of alcohol hand wash.

- Proper Technique: Use the correct duration and procedure of hand washing.

B. Personal Protective Equipment (PPE):

- Gloves: Use sterile gloves during procedures touching clean surfaces or items.

- Gowns and Masks: Wear sterile gowns and masks whenever required to avoid contamination.

C. Sterile Field:

- Definition: Surface or designated area considered microbiologically safe.

- Creation: Establish a sterile field using sterile drapes or covers.

- Maintenance: To ensure no contamination occurs, do not reach over or lean onto the sterile field.

D. Sterile Supplies:

- Handling: Sterilize the gloves before touching any of the medical instruments.

- Presentation: Use aseptic techniques in open sterile supplies.

E. No-Touch Technique:

- Principle: Avoid unnecessary contact with sterile things or objects.

- Instrument Transfer: Move sterile materials using forceps or other appropriate devices.

3. Common Sterile Procedures:

A. Surgical Procedures:

- Preparation: Clean up of surgical sites through the use of antiseptic solutions.

- Dropping: Use intra-operative sterile drapes to demarcate the area of surgery.

B. Central Line Insertion:
- Full Barrier Precautions: Put on a sterile gown, gloves, mask, and cap.
- Aseptic Site Preparation: Clean the insertion site using antiseptic solutions.

C. Wound Dressing Changes:
- Aseptic Technique: Ensure you follow the aseptic technique to curb infection spread.
- Sterile Dressings: Sterile dressings and materials should be used during the process.

4. Sterile Field Maintenance:
- Awareness: Ensure that you are always on guard and watch out for any compromises on the sterile field.

- Immediate Response: Ensure immediate action is taken concerning contamination or a breach.

- Limit Movement: Movements around the sterile fields should be minimized in order not to cause contaminations.

5. Sterile Gloving and Gowning:
- Proper Sequence: Use standard steps for putting on and taking off sterilized gloves as well as garments.

- Avoiding Contamination: Pay attention to the movements and make sure you don't contaminate by mistake while doing so.

6. Post-Procedure Care:
- Disposal of Contaminated Items: Put contaminated materials into suitable containers.
- Hand Hygiene: Wash hands properly after wearing gloves during sterile procedures.

7. Training and Education:

- Continuous Training: Educate and train regularly health care providers in maintaining sterile techniques.

- Competency Assessment: Ensure continuous evaluation and verification of healthcare provider competence in sterile procedures.

8. Documentation

- Record Keeping: Sterile procedures for the document must stipulate the date of occurrence, timeline, and the names of people who were there during that particular time of sterile procedure.

- Monitoring and Audits: Perform routine audits, and assessments on sterile technique adherence.

4.3 Disposal Of Sharps

1. Definition:

- Sharps: Puncturing instruments or sharp objects like needles, syringes, lancets, and scalpels.

- Disposal: Safe dispensing of the sharps to avoid injuries and infections.

2. Importance of Proper Disposal:

- Prevention of Injuries: Minimizes the danger of needle-stick injuries for healthcare workers and others.

- Infection Control: Decreases the likelihood of transmitting contagious pathogens.

- Environmental Protection: It helps in safeguarding the community and the environment against hazardous waste.

3. Regulatory Guidelines:

- OSHA (Occupational Safety and Health Administration): Offers a roadmap for the safe handling and disposal of sharps within healthcare facilities.

- CDC (Centers for Disease Control and Prevention): Gives guidelines on what to put on a sharps disposal as part of infection control.

4. Sharps Containers:
- Purpose: Sharps boxes or specific containers for collecting and disposal of sharps waste.
- Material: Impenetrable and impervious, to protect against the chance of incidental exposure.
- Color Coding: Color coded for example, and usually labeled using biohazard sign.

5. Disposal Procedures:

A. In Healthcare Settings:
- Point of Use: Immediately dispose of sharps in designated containers after use.
- Never Recap: Do not recap needles, just throw each of them in the sharp container.

B. Home Healthcare:

- Personal Sharps Containers: Utilize containers intended for use at home.

- Local Regulations: Comply with the appropriate regulations for domestic sharps management.

6. Needle Destruction Devices:

- Purpose: Devices that automatically and/or electrically crush needles and make them unusable upon destruction.

- Supplement to Containers: Safety used on top of sharp containers.

7. Mail-Back Programs:

- Availability: Mail-back options are also available in some areas and people can dispatch used sharps containers safely.

- Convenience: Gives an option to non-local home users of waste management means.

8. Community Drop-Off Locations:

- Pharmacies and Clinics: Some pharmacies and healthcare institutions also allow the disposal of used sharps.

- Public Awareness: Promote safe disposal at community drop sites.

9. Educational Initiatives:

- Patient Education: Educate patients and the public on the need for correct sharps disposal.

- Safe Practices: Encourage safe practices at home and in health care to minimize injury incidents.

10. Professional Responsibility:

- Healthcare Workers: Comply with institutions' procedures for sharps disposal.

- Leadership Support: Promote safety awareness and make suitable arrangements for appropriate waste management.

11. Environmental Considerations:

- Waste Segregation: Promote proper separation of sharps waste from other forms of waste.

- Waste Management Practices: Ensure that you dispose of the medical waste as per local waste management regulations.

12. Monitoring and Compliance:

- Audits and Inspections: Periodically audit adherence to sharps disposal procedures.

- Continuous Improvement: Introduce the feedback mechanism and continuous quality improvement strategies to improve safety.

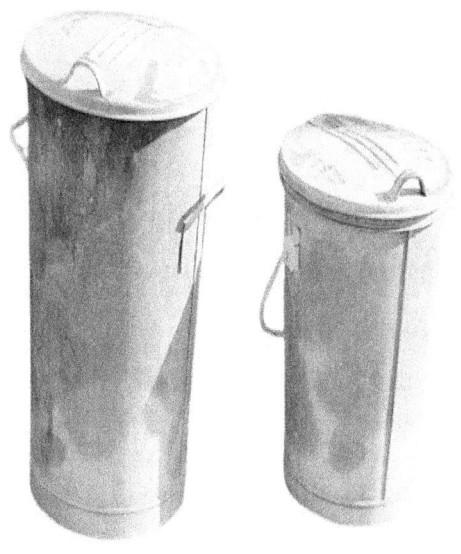

Waste manage can

CHAPTER 5: PATIENT ASSESSMENT

5.1 Preparing The Patient

1. Patient Communication:
- Explanation: inform the patient about the planned procedures.
- Informed Consent: Obtain informed consent from the patient, explaining to them the aim, possible adverse effects, and advantages of the procedure.

2. Informed Consent:
- Process: Provide essential information and seek written or verbal consent from the patient after that.
- Documentation: ensure that the process of informed consent is documented in the patient record.

3. Physical Preparation:

- Patient Comfort: Make sure that a patient is comfortable and well-informed on what he's going through in the environment.

- Positioning: Place the patient in the proper position based on the procedure considerations and the patient's ease.

4. Verification of Patient Identity:

- Checklist: Verify the patient's identity using a two-identifier system (e.g., name and date of birth).

- Patient Engagement: This should be a mutual process that involves the patient to help improve accuracy.

5. Medical History Review:

- Current Medications: Assess the patient's present medications for allergy reaction as well as possible contraindications.

- Health Conditions: Determine the state of general well-being of a patient and any other underlying illnesses.

6. Allergy Assessment:

- Allergies: Check on all allergies known and take all measures possible to avert allergens.

- Contrast Media: If applicable to certain procedures, ask about allergies to the contrast media.

7. Fasting Instructions:

- NPO (Nothing by Mouth): If necessary, give directions on fasting before the process.

- Medication Exceptions: Give specific directions for taking some medicines along with a drink of water.

8. Mental and Emotional Support:

- Patient Anxiety: Effective communication, including being able to understand oneself and others will help address and alleviate patient anxiety.

- Support Person: In cases where the patient, is comfortable with a support person present, allow one to be there.

9. Pain Management:

- Pre-procedure Analgesia: Give painkillers as necessary per physician's orders.

- Pain Assessment: Determine their present or baseline pain scores and answer the questions raised.

10. Communication with the Care Team:

- Team Briefing: Inform the healthcare personnel about the patient's history, allergies, and special considerations.

- Clarifications: Answer the challenges posed to the patients or their families.

11. Pre-procedure Checklist:

- Verify Equipment: Check whether required tools, machines, and other essentials are readily available in good conditions of serviceability.

- Documentation: Ensure completion of the necessary paperwork and prior procedure checklists.

12. Patient Privacy and Dignity:

- Modesty: Provide proper draping and privacy hence respecting their modesty.

- Clear Communication: Provide clarity by explaining in detail each step of the preparation process to the patient.

13. Post-procedure Instructions:

- Aftercare: Give detailed instructions on aftercare procedures such as the restrictions, medication, and possibly follow-up consultations.

- Emergency Contact: Make sure that there is ready access to the emergency telephone numbers for the patient.

14. Emotional Support Post-Procedure:

- Debriefing: Provide an additional consultation to discuss the possible psychological after-effects of the procedure.

- Follow-up: Set further appointments based on the progress of healing and monitoring.

5.2 Assessing veins for IV injections.

1. Patient Assessment:

- Medical History: Review your patient's history and note any issues related to vein choice such as previous operations and existing chronic illnesses.

- Allergies and Sensitivities: Identify allergies or sensitivities that may affect IV solution and IV equipment selection.

2. Informed Consent:

- Communication: Inform the patient about why you are performing an IV injection and how it is done.

- Consent: Give the patient detailed information about the IV procedure and make sure they understand its potential risks and benefits, seeking their informed consent.

3. Gather Equipment:

- IV Catheter: Choose an appropriate catheter size depending on the purpose and patient's conditions.

- Tourniquet: To enhance blood vessel visualization, prepare a tourniquet.

- Sterile Gloves and Supplies: Sanitize all equipment before commencing.

4. Patient Positioning:

- Comfort: Make sure the patient is comfortable and feeling at ease.

- Accessibility: Select an area that makes it easier to locate likely injection sites.

5. Vein Selection Criteria:

- Vein Visibility: Choose a vein that is both visible and palpable.

- Vein Size: Take into account the size of the vein concerning the catheter size.

- Condition of Vein: Evaluate the quality of the vein in parts free from damage or inflammatory signs.

6. Common Sites for IV Placement:

- Cephalic Vein: The location is in the forearm, at the radial side.

- Basilic Vein: Located on the ulnar side of the wrist.
- Median Cubital Vein: Situated in the antecubital fossa.
- Dorsal Hand Veins: However especially for individual situations like when you couldn't get in other sites.

7. Assess Vein Resilience:
- Elasticity: Select a distended vein with retractive ability.
- Depth: Pay attention to the vein's depth so that you do not try to find too deep or superficial veins.

8. Assess Vein Fragility:
- Fragile Veins: When you have patients who are advanced in age and/or have diseases that could cause their veins to bruise faster, be careful.
- Assess Capillary Refill: Assess capillary refill for blood flow assessment.

9. Tourniquet Application:

- Purpose: Improve the visualization of the veins and promote painless access.

- Location: Place the tourniquet distal to the planned injection point.

- Duration: Use tourniquets for only a short time to prevent complications.

10. Warm Compress:

- Comfort Measure: Use a warm compress to facilitate vasodilation at the chosen site.

- Vein Dilation: The veins are also more visible in situations where there is a warmer temperature since they widen.

11. Patient Education:

- Explanation: Teach the patient about the process, what they might feel during it, and the value of keeping still during an injection.

- Ongoing Communication: Ensure regular communication with the patient as a process.

12. Document the Assessment:

- Record Keeping: Record the results of the assessment such as a selected vein, difficulties experienced, and patient reactions.

Injections - Ensure Compliance: Adhere to institutional documentation protocols.

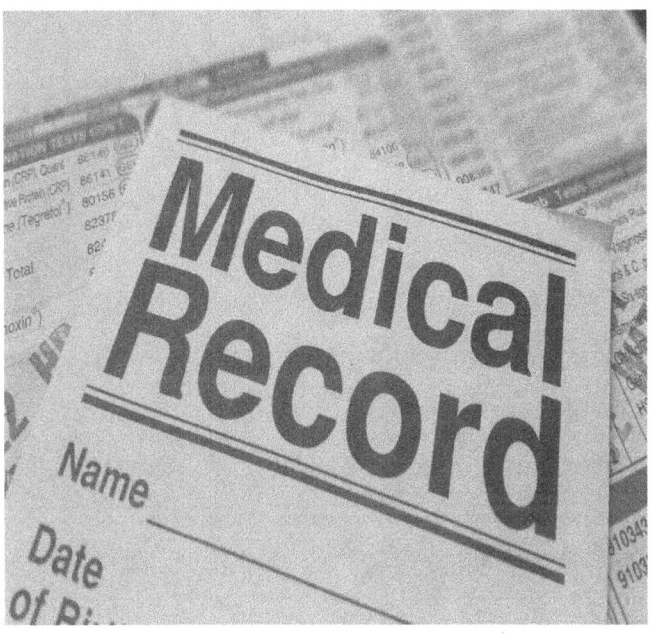

5.3. Assessment of muscles for IM injections

1. Patient Assessment:

- Health History: Discuss the patient's health history to identify any conditions or factors that will influence muscle integrity or the choice of injection sites.

- Allergies: Also, confirm any allergy, especially medication that can be injected IM.

2. Informed Consent:

- Communication: In simple terms, elucidate why, what are its benefits, and how it is likely to compromise the individual.

- Consent: Informed consent of the patient or his/her legal representative.

3. Gather Equipment:

- Syringe and Needle: Choose the proper syringe and size of a needle according to the features of a patient and the intended area of injection.

- Alcohol Swabs: Maintain sterility when preparing an injection site.
- Medication: Verify the correct drug and dose ordered for IM injection.

4. Patient Positioning:
- Comfort: Make sure that the patient feels comfortable throughout.
- Accessible Site: Find an open area that will make it possible to penetrate the targeted site with ease.

5. Common IM Injection Sites:
- Deltoid Muscle: The Deltoid muscle is located in the upper arm.
- Ventrogluteal Muscle: Situated in the hip area.
- Vastus Lateralis: Found in the thigh.

6. Assessment of Muscle Mass:
- Palpation: Measure the muscle mass through gentle palpation of the selected injection area.
- Comparison: If possible, consider comparing between the two sides' muscle masses.

7. Muscle Integrity:

- No Signs of Inflammation: Refrain from injecting into sites that are inflamed, red, and swollen.

- Scarring or Lesions: Feel for any scars or nodules in muscle tissues.

8. Local Anatomical Landmarks:

- Deltoid Muscle: Point out the acromion process and instill it in the middle.

- Ventrogluteal Muscle: Identify these sites such as the greater trochanter, anterior superior iliac spine, and iliac crest.

- Vastus Lateralis: Inject in the middle of the divided thirds of the thigh.

9. Patient Factors:

- Age: Take into account the different influences based on age including muscle growth and patient compliance.

- Weight: Considering adipose tissue thickness and muscle mass adjustments of needle length.

10. Aspiration Check:
- Purpose: Aspirate before injecting and ensure that the needle isn't in a blood vessel.
- No Blood Return: Check for reversal of pulses before giving this medicine.

11. Patient Education:
- Explanation: Inform the patient about what happens during an IM injection, the different feelings that may be experienced, and why it is necessary to hold still.
- Post-Injection Care: Indicate directions for precautionary measures following injection and probable aftermaths.

12. Document the Assessment:
- Record Keeping: Make notes of all findings regarding the assessments, the chosen injection point, problems encountered, as well as reactions by the patient involved.
- Ensure Compliance: Adhere to institutional documentation protocols.

CHAPTER 6: IV INJECTION PROCEDURE

6. 1 Selecting the IV Site

1. Patient Assessment:

- Medical History: Take a look at the patient's medical history as it relates to what could influence IV site selection such as previous surgeries or chronic conditions.

- Allergies and Sensitivities: Ascertain whether there are any allergy-related considerations, such as preferred infusion fluids and devices of administration.

2. Informed Consent:

- Communication: Talk to the patient about why he should be injected with an IV and how it will be done.

- Consent: Secure informed consent for IV procedure and make sure that a patient comprehends possible risks and benefits.

3. Gather Equipment:

- IV Catheter: Choose a suitable catheter size based on the selected purpose of the use and patient attributes.

- Tourniquet: Place a tourniquet above the injury to increase vein visibility.

- Sterile Gloves and Supplies: Sterilize all required equipment so as not to spread any infections.

4. Patient Positioning:

- Comfort: Make sure the patient is feeling comfortable and relaxed.

- Accessibility: Ensure you select an easy-to-inject area on which position.

5. Vein Selection Criteria:

- Vein Visibility: Pick out a vein that will be very visible and palpable.

- Vein Size: Think about the size of the vein for comparison with the catheter size.

- Condition of Vein: Determine the viability of the vein, and avoid regions exhibiting evidence of swelling or disruption.

6. Common Sites for IV Placement:
- Cephalic Vein: It lies on the outer aspect of the arm.
- Basilic Vein: It is situated at the medial aspect of the forearm.
- Median Cubital Vein: Situated in the antecubital fossa.

7. Assess Vein Resilience:
- Elasticity: Select an elastic vessel that would easily expand and contract as well.
- Depth: Think about the length of the vein and how it is not too superficial nor extremely deep.

8. Assess Vein Fragility:
- Fragile Veins: Ensure you are extra careful when dealing with old patients or those who have

conditions that increase the likelihood of bruising and infiltration.

- Assess Capillary Refill: Assess the capillary refill to determine vascular function.

9. Tourniquet Application:

- Purpose: Improve visibility of venous structures, and facilitate venipuncture.

- Location: Place this in proximity to the point of insertion.

- Duration: Apply a tourniquet for a brief period only to prevent complications.

10. Warm Compress:

- Comfort Measure: Promote vasodilation by introducing a warm compress in the targeted region.

- Vein Dilation: Higher temperatures may help widen and highlight veins.

patient

11. Patient Education:

- Explanation: Explain to the patient about the process, possible feelings the patient could experience, and the need for immobility during the insertion.

- Ongoing Communication: Ensure you communicate openly with your patients during the whole procedure.

12. Document the Assessment:

- Record Keeping: Record the assessments that are made such as the selected vein with any difficulties encountered and patient comments.

- Ensure Compliance: Adhere to institutional documentation protocols.

6.2 Intravenous (IV)Insertion Techniques

1. Hand Hygiene and Personal Protective Equipment:

- Hand Washing: The provider must wash the hands thoroughly before the process.

- Gloves: Ensure that sterile gloves are always on to have an aseptic environment.

2. Patient Positioning:

- Comfort: Position your desired limb comfortably away from the patient such that it is stretched and supported.

- Accessibility: Select a convenient spot that will guide the way directly to the chosen entry point.

3. Vein Assessment and Selection:

- Palpation: Assess the size, elasticity, and depth of the vein by gently palpating it.

- Visual Inspection: Verify visualization of the vein and select an area void of symptoms indicating inflammation/damage.

4. Tourniquet Application:
- Purpose: Improve the visibility of veins, making venipuncture easy.
- Location: Tie the tourniquet as close to the chosen puncture point as possible.
- Duration: The tourniquets should be limited in time of use since prolonged exposure may cause complications.

5. Skin Preparation:
- Alcohol Swabbing: Perform an alcohol hand rub on the chosen insertion site, moving roundly.
- Allow Drying: Ensure that there is complete drying of the skin and then continue.

6. Anchoring the Vein:
- Tension: Provide gentle traction to the surrounding skin to stabilize the selected vein.

- Prevent Vein Rolling: Prevent rolling of the vein during the process of insertion.

7. Needle Insertion:

- Angle: For superficial veins, insert the needle at an angle of 15-30 degrees and use a 30-45-degree angle for deeper ones.

- Smooth Insertion: Insert the needle into the vein using a smooth, controlled motion. - Aspiration Check: Aspiration is done to confirm that the catheter has reached the atrium of the heart when blood returns are seen and proceeding ahead.

8. Catheter Advancement:

- Insertion Angle: Rotate the needle to any necessary angle while still using it.

- Catheter Thread: Move the needle forward and advance the catheter into the vein without any loss of needle control.

9. Needle Withdrawal:

- Withdrawal Technique: Slowly and smoothly withdraw the needle leaving the catheter in place.

- Visual Confirmation: Ensure that the catheter is placed in the vein.

10. Catheter Securement:

- Adhesive Securement: Secure the catheter using adhesive securement devices.

- Avoid over-tightening: To be secure but not overtighten to avoid complications.

11. Hub and Flush:

- Hub Connection: Securely connect the catheter hub to the IV tubing.

- Saline Flush: It helps ensure the patency of the catheter by flushing it with a saline solution.

12. Dressing Application:

- Sterile Dressing: Cover the insertion site with a sterile dressing.

- Transparency: Select a see-through bandage for continuity.

13. Post-Insertion Monitoring:

- Assessment: Check the patient for any symptoms that may indicate complications such as infiltration or phlebitis.
- Documentation: Describe in detail the procedure steps like the site, catheter size, and any complications.

14. Patient Education:

- Explanation: Inform the patient about the IV line; tell them to expect certain feelings in the area; emphasize that they should notify the nurse if they experience pain in the area.
- Comfort Measures: Provide comfort measures and reassurance.

15. Disposal of Sharps and Waste:

- Sharps Container: Place the needle and other sharps into a safe sharps container for disposal.

- Waste Disposal: Waste management should be done in line with institutional guidelines.

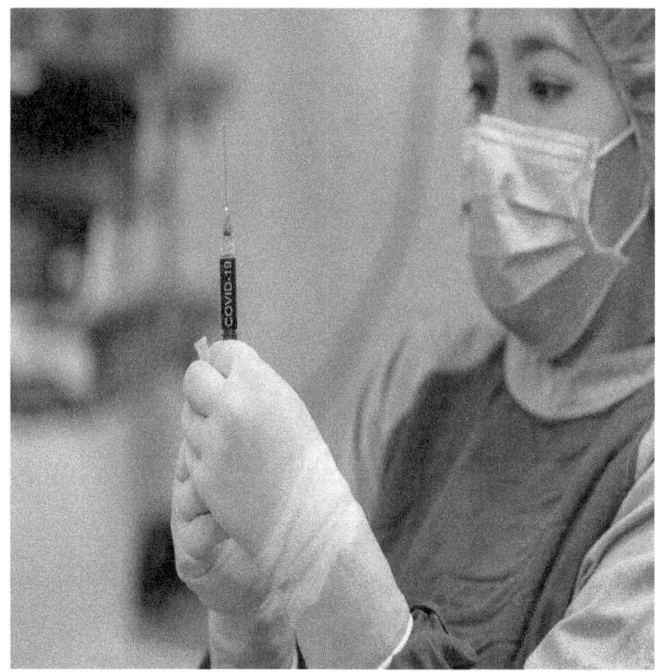

6. 3 Monitoring For Complications Monitor

1. Immediate Post-Insertion Assessment:
- Patient Comfort: Determine, if the patient is comfortable with it and discuss any issues or worries that have emerged.
- Dressing Integrity: Check that the dressing is properly intact.

2. Vital Sign Monitoring:
- Frequency: Keep vigilant of them, especially upon insertion in the early stages.
- Signs of Instability: Watch out for hypotension, tachycardia, and other markers of circulatory decompensation.

3. Site Inspection:
- Color and Temperature: Check the surrounding temperature and skin of the insertion site.
- Swelling or Redness: Check for any evidence of swelling, redness, or inflammation.

4. Infiltration Assessment:

- Palpation: Palpate gently around the IV site for swelling, hardness, and coldness.

- Patient Complaints: Note all pains and discomforts in the area.

5. Phlebitis Evaluation:

- Redness and Warmth: Inspect for redness; warmth along or tenderness over the vein course.

- Patient Reports: Note down any signs of pain, discomfort, or irritation while keeping up records.

6. Catheter Patency Check:

- Flushing: To facilitate flushing, check if there are any obstructions or resistance.

- Blood Return: Ensure blood return occurs during flushing.

7. Systemic Complications:

- Fever: Look out for symptoms like fever; this could mean the presence of systemic infection.

- Chills: Inspect cases of chilliness, as they could be linked to infections.

8. Assess for Hematoma:
- Swelling and Discoloration: At the insertion site look out for signs of hematoma formation.
- Palpation: Lightly press around there to feel for anything abnormal like a mass.".

9. Continuous Monitoring for Allergic Reactions:
- Observation: It is important to observe the patient for any sign of an allergic reaction like a rash, Itchiness, or respiratory distress.
- Immediate Intervention: Ensure quick intervention, in case of an allergy attack.

10. Neurovascular Assessment:
- Circulation: Evaluate peripheral circulation at the site of the IV insertion into a limb.
- Sensation: Test sensation by asking the person whether they experience tingling or numbness.

11. Documentation:

- Detailed Record Keeping: Record each assessment, intervention, and patient's response.

- Timeliness: Document all complications on time and ensure that follow-ups are done with due accuracy.

12. Patient Education:

- Signs to Report: Inform the patient on what signs or symptoms they need to report including worsening of pain, swelling, or redness.

- Contact Information: Give details on where you can get help in case of complications/concerns.

13. Follow-Up Assessments:

- Scheduled Checks: Make arrangements for periodic follow-up assessments.

- Reassess and Document: Review the IV site as well as the patient's condition at every visit.

14. Collaboration with Healthcare Team:

- Communication: Inform the medical team of observed complications when they happen.

- Collaborative Decision-Making: Make a joint decision on the catheter's removal or some alternatives.

15. Policies and Protocols:

- Adherence: Monitor complications according to the institutions' policies and procedures.

- Reporting: Immediately report any complication through the provided channels.

Chapter 7: IM INJECTION PROCEDURE PROCEDURE

7. 1. choose Intramuscular (IM) injection site

1. Patient Assessment:

- Health History: Check the health record of the patient including allergies, medical problems, and other reactions towards injections.

- Allergies and Sensitivities: Any existing drugs and allergies will also need to be considered, especially those that might be injected as a form of a drug dosage.

2. Informed Consent:

- Communication: Explain to the patient how it works, why he or she needs it, and what risks come with it.

- Consent: Ensure that you have obtained informed consent from the patient's guardian.

3. Gather Equipment:
- Syringe and Needle: Choose a suitable syringe and needle size depending on the features of the patient and the site for the injecting process.
- Alcohol Swabs: Sterilize the environment of your injection/site preparation.
- *Medication: Verify the given medication and the dosage for IM injection are accurate.

4. Patient Positioning:
- Comfort: The patient must be feeling comfortable and as much as possible at ease.
- Accessible Site: Select an accessible place, from which it is possible to enter a certain injection spot.

5. Common IM Injection Sites:
- Deltoid Muscle: Located in the upper arm.
- Ventrogluteal Muscle: Situated in the hip area.
- Vastus Lateralis: Found in the thigh.

6. Assessment of Muscle Mass:

- Palpation: To assess muscle mass, gently palpate at the intended injection site.

- Comparison: If applicable, consider comparing the muscle mass between the two sides.

7. Muscle Integrity:

- No Signs of Inflammation: It is necessary to avoid using areas with inflammation, reddening, or edema for injection purposes.

- Scarring or Lesions: Determine scarring and muscular lesions.

8. Local Anatomical Landmarks:

- Deltoid Muscle: Locate the acromion process and inject into the mid-third.

- Ventrogluteal Muscle: You need to identify the greater trochanter, anterior superior iliac spine, and the iliac crest to correctly select a site.

- Vastus Lateralis: Split the thigh into three parts and then inject it in its midpoint part.

9. Patient Factors:

- Age: Take into account the patient's muscular development and how cooperative they are.

- Weight: Set needle length according to tissues' thickness, and muscles' mass.

10. Aspiration Check:
- Purpose: Aspirate before injecting to confirm that a needle does not pierce through blood vessels.
-vesselsood Return: Make sure there is no retrograde flow of blood before injecting the drug.

11. Patient Education:
- Explanation: Explain the IM injection procedure to the patient, the sensations associated with it, and the importance of being still during the puncture.
- Post-Injection Care: Describe post-injection care plans and possible side-effects.

12. Document the Assessment:
- Record Keeping: Record your observations such as the injection site and difficulties experienced while injecting as well as any complaints by the patients during and after the procedure.
- Ensure Compliance: Adhere to institutional documentation protocols.

7.2 Insertion Depth and Angle Need.

1. Needle Insertion Depth:

- Deltoid Muscle:

- Adults: Hold the needle perpendicular to the deltoid and insert it.

- Children and Adolescents: Ninety degrees is usually appropriate because of a thinner muscle layer.

- Ventrogluteal Muscle:

- Adults and Children: Make sure that you insert the needle perpendicularly.

- Vastus Lateralis Muscle:

- Adults and Children: Holding the needle at a right angle.

2. Needle Insertion Angle:

- Deltoid Muscle:

- Adults: Place the needle at a 90-degree angle right through.

- Children and Adolescents: In this case, a typical inclination is approximately 90 degrees because of a thinner muscle layer.

- Ventrogluteal Muscle:
- Adults and Children: Ensure that you insert the needle on a perpendicular basis.

- Vastus Lateralis Muscle:
- Adults and Children: Put the needle into the skin at a right angle.

3. Considerations for Angle Adjustment:
- Adipose Tissue Thickness: The angle of the needle penetration might need to be changed in a patient with much adipose tissue so that a needle contacts the muscle layer.
- Pediatric Patients: The length of the needle might be shorter in some cases involving pediatric patients and then the angle can also be adjusted.

4. Depth Guidelines:

- Deltoid Muscle:

- Depth: Make sure that you puncture the muscle appropriately by inserting the needle completely.

- Ventrogluteal Muscle:

- Depth: Make sure that the needle is fully inserted into the muscle.engine:

- Vastus Lateralis Muscle:

- Depth: Ensure proper penetration of the muscle by inserting the needle to its full length.

5. Avoiding Subcutaneous Injection:

- Angle and Depth: Be extra cautious about the angle and depth as it could end up injecting the medicine into connective tissue unintentionally.

6. Assessing for Proper Placement:

- Patient Response: Pay attention to the patient who may feel unwell with the injection.

- Aspiration Check: Confirm that aspirating shows no blood back then inject the drug.

7. Needle Withdrawal:
- Smooth Withdrawal: Gently pull out the needle to prevent tissue damage.
- Observe for Bleeding: Observe for bleeding and/or hematoma development at the injection site.

8. Documentation:
- Record Needle Details: Record the gauge size, the amount of penetration, and the angles involved in the injection.
- Patient Response: Record whether or not the patient responds, or any complications if they occur.

9. Adherence to Institutional Protocols:
- Consistency: Adhere to institutional protocols on needle penetration depths and angles as well as other health requirements, such as sterility of the equipment.
- Regular Training: Provide continuous education on appropriate injection skills for healthcare professionals.

7.3 Z-track method for minimizing medication leakage during IM injection.

1. Patient Preparation:

- Explanation: Explain clearly to the patient the Z-track method indicating how it minimizes drug leakage as well as pain during administration.

- Informed Consent: Seek the informed consent of the patient first.

2. Gather Equipment:

- Syringe and Needle: Choose a suitable syringe and needle dependent on the drugs and patients.

- Alcohol Swabs: Prepare clean injection sites.

- Medication: Ensure that the medication was correctly prescribed for IM administration.

3. Choose an Injection Site:
- Common Sites:
- Ventrogluteal Muscle: A thicker muscle layer is often preferred.

- Vastus Lateralis Muscle: To be used on pediatric cases in particular, also when ventral lateral opening is not possible.
- Deltoid Muscle: For some drugs used on adult patients.

4. Patient Positioning:
- Accessibility: Set up the patient in a way that makes it easy for one to access the designated injection area without any difficulties
- Comfort: Ensure that the patient is comfortable in a suitable position for the selected site.

5. Z-Track Technique:
Locate the Site: Select an appropriate injection site that can be used safely, for instance, the ventrolateral muscle.
- Skin Displacement: Skin should be pulled laterally so that it makes an up Z displacing it from the underlying muscle.
- Needle Insertion: Stick the needle vertically in the muscle through the displaced skin.

- Aspiration Check: Draw air into a syringe and aim to avoid inserting the needle into a blood vessel.
- Medication Administration: It should be administered gradually.

6. Maintain Skin Displacement:
- Throughout Injection: To avoid backtracking in the needle track during the injection, leave the skin displaced all along.

7. Needle Withdrawal:
- Smooth Withdrawal: Holding the skin in a displace, remove the needle smooth and steady.
- Allow Skin to Return: After the withdrawal the needle withdraws, it releases the displaced skin.

8. Assess for Bleeding or Leakage:
- Observation: Ascertain the injection site for blood leak and drug escape.
- Apply Gentle Pressure: If required, press on a sterile pad at the site of bleeding using gentle pressure to reduce it.

9. Patient Comfort Measures:

- Post-Injection Care: Give directions on the need for post-injection care and possibly comfort for one's self if necessary.

- Address Discomfort: Answer all questions and address any discomfort the patient may be having.

10. Documentation:

- Record Details: Record and document the site, the needle used, and the encountered complications using the z-method.

- Patient Response: Record the patients' responses as well as all the related complaints.

11. Adherence to Institutional Protocols:

- Consistency: Adhere to institutional guidelines and protocols on the Z-track method.

- Regular Training: Healthcare professionals should have their regular training on correct injectable methods.

CHAPTER 8: MEDICATION ADMINISTRATION

8.1 Guidelines For Dilution, And Mixing Iv And Im Intra Prescription Drugs.

1. Medication Compatibility Assessment:

- Review Prescribing Information: Make sure that you review the product label for compatibility of diluents and other drugs.

- Consult Pharmacy or Formulary: For special dilution guidelines refer to the pharmacy or formulary.

2. Use Sterile Technique:

- Equipment and Environment: In the event of infection, ensure the equipment is sterilized as well as the environment.

3. Diluent Selection:

- Compatibility: The chosen diluent should be appropriate for the drug, and the proposed route of its administration (for example saline for IV drugs).

- Manufacturer Recommendations: Observe any recommendation provided by the manufacturer regarding the choice of a diluent.

4. Calculations:

- Dosage and Volume: Calculate the specified dose and volume from the prescribed concentration (end concentration).

- Labeling: Ensure you label your diluted solution with the accurate medication name, concentration, and date of expiration.

5. Mixing Procedure:

- Gentle Mixing: To ensure that foam does not form, the mixture should be gentle with either inversion or stirring from side to side.

- Avoid Contamination: Mixing should be done under cleanliness conditions as mixing equipment should be sterile.

6. Compatibility with IV Fluids:
- Verify Compatibility: Ensure that it is compatible with the selected IV fluid like normal saline or dextrose.
- Avoid Precipitation: Make sure to check for any precipitation and discoloration as these may point to incompatibility.

7. Check for Particulate Matter:
- Visual Inspection: Ensure that the medicine is free from particles as well as unusual colors before and after dilution.
- Discard if Necessary: If there's particulate matter, do not use that solution as it was contaminated and make a new one.

8. Sequential Mixing of Medications:

- Check Compatibility: Before any mix of different medications, ascertain their compatibility when combined.

- Sequential Mixing: Dissolve individually and adequately mix the drugs, making sure the solution contains the appropriate amount of water.

9. Time Constraints:

- Follow Recommendations: Comply with the time limitations defined by the medicatmanufacturer'surer instructions or the institution's guidelines for the stability of the solution after dilution.

10. Labeling:

- Clear Identification: The final diluted solution must be clearly labeled to indicate the drug name, expiry date, and any other relevant data.

- *Patient Identification: Patient-specific information should be provided to avoid drug administration errors.

11. Storage Conditions:

- Temperature and Light: Keep the diluted solution under the required temperature and protection from light as required by the guidelines.

- Duration: As per the institution's policy, throw out any solutions that are past the expiration date or are leftover.

12. Documentation:

- Record Details: Document each step of dilution and mixings (including calculations, diluents, and any problems).

- Verify Orders: Check if the dilution conforms to the doctor's instructions.

13. Adherence to Institutional Protocols:

- Consistency: Dilute or mix according to the standard operational procedure.

- Regular Training: Conduct frequent educative programs for health care professionals about correct diluting and mixing methods.

8.2 Administering Medication: IV Push and IV Infusion

1. Patient Assessment:

- Vital Signs: Take vital signs to make certain that the patient will be stable for administration of the drug.

- Medical History: Assess the patient's past medical record, allergy profile, and current medications.

2. Informed Consent:

- Communication: Emphasize the importance of clearly explaining the medication administration procedure to the patient.

- Consent: To get informed consent of a patient or his/her legal representative.

3. Gather Equipment:

- IV Catheter: Ensure that the IV catheter is well placed.

- Syringe and Needle: Choose the suitable syringe and needle for IV push or infusion.

- Medication: Checking that the right medicine and dosage are given.

4. IV Push Administration:
- Flush the Line: Ensure that your IV line is patent before the IV push with a compatible infused solution.
- Administer Slowly: Give the drug slowly in accord with infusion rates as specified.
- Observe for Reactions: Ensure to observe any negative reactions as you administer.

5. IV Push Considerations:
- Compatibility: Verify that the drug is compatible with the IV line and other solutions.
- Maximum Rate: Avoid complications hence comply with the highest recommended infusion rate.

6. IV Infusion Administration:

- Dilution: Diluting the drug as per institution protocols should be done if required.

- Infusion Pump: Utilizing an infusion pump for controlled and accurate administration.

- Monitor Infusion Rate: This should be done regularly and change the infusion rate accordingly.

7. IV Infusion Considerations:

- Site Assessment: Check for any signs of infiltration or phlebitis at the IV site while still infusion is ongoing.

- Compatibility with IV Fluids: Always try to make the IV fluid compatible to avoid precipitation or incompatibility problems.

8. Compatibility Checks:

- Medication Compatibility: Ascertain appropriateness alongside other co-administered drugs.

- IV Fluid Compatibility: Ensure that the prescribed IV fluid is compatible.

9. Monitoring During Administration:

- Vital Signs: Monitor vital signs during the infusion administration, especially if it concerns an adverse reaction.

- Patient Comfort: Listen to the patient's complaints and ease their discomfort.

10. Documentation:

- Record Details: Include details on the medicine, for example, medication name, dose, route, time, and any noted patient reactions.

- Infusion Pump Settings: The document should record pump set-up parameters and changes that occurred while infusing.

11. Post-Administration Monitoring:

- Observation: Check on the patient for late side effects and state changes following the drug intake.

- Documentation: Conduct a follow-up assessment on documentation, as well as intervention if required.

12. Adherence to Institutional Protocols:

- Consistency: Observe the institution's policy on IV push and infusion.

- Regular Training: Provide periodic educational sessions to all healthcare professionals regarding appropriate methods of giving medications.

8. 3 Intramuscular (IM) Injection Technique

1. Patient Preparation:

Explanation: Explain in clear terms how the IM injection is done and clarify any doubts the patient could have on issues concerning his or her health, as well as reassure him/her about the safety of the injection.

- Informed Consent: The healthcare provider should obtain informed consent of the patient or the patient's legal representative.

2. Gather Equipment:

- Syringe and Needle: Choose the most suitable syringe and needle gauge considering different patient attributes, as well as the point of injection.

- Alcohol Swabs: Safeguard appropriate sterile conditions during injection site preparation.

- Medication: Verify the right medication and dosage meant for IM administration.

3. Choose an Injection Site:

- Common Sites:

- Deltoid Muscle: Located in the upper arm.

- Ventrogluteal Muscle: Situated in the hip area.

- Vastus Lateralis: Found in the thigh.

4. Patient Positioning:

- Comfort: Make the patient as comfortable and comfortable as possible.

- Accessible Site: Select a convenient spot for administering an injection.

5. Skin Preparation:

- Alcohol Swabbing: Circle-wise cleansing of the injection site utilizing an alcohol swabbed.

- Allow Drying: Wait for the entire skin to fully dry before you move on.

6. Needle Insertion:

- Angle: To begin with, insert the needle at a right angle for most adults and older children. Thin people and children can adjust as shown in degrees 45 or 60.

- Smooth Insertion: Inject slowly and smoothly into a muscle.

- Aspiration Check: Suck back ensuring that the needle is not in a blood vessel before giving the medicine.

7. Medication Administration:

- Slow and Steady: Give the medicine as slow and sure method as possible to avoid pain and limit the injury.

- Patient Comfort: Educate the patient to relax while giving for less tension.

8. Needle Withdrawal:

- Smooth Withdrawal: Minimize tissue trauma by withdrawing the needle smoothly and steadily.

- Pressure Application: Use a sterilized gauze pad to place very light pressure on the injection wound area and minimal bleeding after application of the injection.

9. Assess for Bleeding or Leakage:
- Observation: Check for bleeding or medication leakage on the injection site.
- Apply Gentle Pressure: Put a dry sterile gauze pad over the wound and press gently to reduce bleeding.

10. Post-Injection Care:
- Comfort Measures: Give aftercare post-injection advice which includes the use of warm compresses and nonprescription painkillers if needed.
- Observation: Check on the patient and ensure that there are no delayed reactions or complications.

11. Documentation:
- Record Details: Note down the IM injection information like site, needle gauge, drug used, dose applied, as well as seen side effects.
- Patient Response: Record how the patient responded and any pain experienced.

12. Adherence to Institutional Protocols:
- Consistency: They should follow the protocol of in-institutional procedures that govern IM injection.
- Regular Training: There is a need for regular training of healthcare professionals on correct IM injection techniques.

CHAPTER 9:

DOCUMENTATION AND

RECORD-KEEPING

9.1 charting administration of Medication.

1. Patient Identification:

- Verify Identity: Use at least two patient identifiers such as name and date of birth in confirming the patient's identity.

2. Date and Time:

- Record Administration Time: Ensure that you record the exact date and time that a patient takes his medicine/s.

3. Medication Details:

- Medication Name: identify the name of the medicine given.

- Dosage: Record the exact dosage administered.

- Route of Administration: Describe route(s) of administration(e.g. IV, IM, PO).
- Site: Indicate the injection point for IM or IV drugs.
- Dilution Details: Documenting if possible any process of mixing or dissolution carried out.

4. Administration Method:
- IV Push or Infusion: Was it IV push or infusion?page
- IM Injection: State whether the drug was injected in a muscle.

5. Equipment Details:
- Syringe and Needle: Write down the size of the syringe and needles involved.
- IV Catheter: Catheter size and site for IV medicines.

6. Patient Response:

- Observations: Describe any patient response/reaction as observed during and after dosing.

- Vital Signs: The monitoring should include vital signs taken either before, during, or after administration of medications.

7. Allergies and Adverse Reactions:

- Allergy Documentation: Check if the patient is allergic to anything, especially antibiotics.

- Adverse Reactions: Record any side effects observed in the patient while giving/after giving administration.

8. Patient Education:

- Communication: Document information on all education given about the medication, such as possible adverse side effects or follow-up instructions.

- Patient Understanding: Write a note on the patients' comprehension and acceptance of what has been explained.

9. Nursing Interventions:
- Any Interventions: Any nursing intervention made concerning complication and management of administration.
- Follow-Up Actions: Record all suggested and/or undertaken follow-up actions.

10. Signature:
- Name and Signature: Put your signature and legibly printed name down as the health care provider giving an order.

11. Documentation Completeness:
- Review: Make sure the documentation is thorough; and complies with the hospital's standard practices and procedures.
- Timeliness: After giving the drug, chart administration details.

12. Adherence to Protocols:

- Consistency: adhere to hospital procedures and policies regarding charting of medications.

- Accuracy: Check if all the items are entered correctly and completely.

13. Communication with the Healthcare Team:

- Reporting: Notify the healthcare team immediately in case of the emergence of additional complications or deviation from the plan.

- Collaboration: Share relevant information with other healthcare providers.

9. 2 Monitoring & Reporting Adverse Effects

1. Patient Observation:

- Continuous Monitoring: Always ensure that the patient is being monitored for any reactions during or after the medication administration.

- Vital Signs: Monitor changes in the vital symptoms including pulse rate, blood pressure, breathing rate,e, and body temperature.

2. Specific Adverse Reactions:

- Anticipate Possible Reactions: Always watch out for possible side effects of the particular drug administered.

- Common Reactions: Watch out for the usual side effects like rashes, pruritus, respiratory distress, and any changes in mental state.

3. Allergy Assessment:

- Known Allergies: Check the patient's known allergies before giving the medication.

- Early Signs: Watch out for early signals of allergies like rashes, swellings, and itches.

4. Respiratory Monitoring:
- Breathing Patterns: Any change in breathing pattern such as difficulty breathing or wheeziness.
- Use of Respiratory Monitoring Devices: If there is a need, one should use respiratory monitoring apparatuses.

5. Neurological Assessment:
- Consciousness: Determine the patient's level of awareness and orientation.
- Neurological Signs: Ensure that you monitor for any confusion, dizziness, seizures, or neurological symptoms.

6. Skin Inspection:
- Skin Integrity: Look over the area where the infection is spreading for any rashes, red patches, swellings, or change of color.

- Injection Site: In case of IV or IM administration, watch out for the reaction on the injection site.

7. Gastrointestinal Observations:
- Nausea and Vomiting: Pay attention to signs of nausea and vomiting.
- Abdominal Pain: Check yourself for any abdominal pain and trouble.

8. Immediate Reporting:
- Critical Reactions: In case of any severe or life-threatening adverse reaction, report to your health care provider or call an emergency unit immediately.
- Follow Institutional Protocols: Comply with institutional procedures for reporting significant matters.

9. Documentation:
- Detailed Record Keeping: Record all noted adverse reactions concerning their manifestation

period, level of intensity, as well as applied interventions in a detailed way.

- Use of Adverse Reaction Forms: Fill in and complete any specific adverse reaction forms, as needed.

10. Communication with the Healthcare Team:
- Timely Reporting: Notify the healthcare team as soon as possible about every reported adverse reaction.
- Collaboration: Work together with other healthcare providers towards an extensive response.

11. Follow-Up Monitoring:
- Continuous Observation: Continue assessing the patient for any of the long-lasting and delayed side effects that might occur.
- Scheduled Assessments: Schedule regular assessments of high-risk medications according to institutional guidelines.

12. Patient Education:

- Explanation: Tell the patient which of the expected side effects you have noticed, including the reasons for them and steps required for further care.

- Document Education: Record information on the patient's education received and whether or not they understood it.

13. Adherence to Protocols:

Consistency: Adhere to institutional regulations and procedures for tracking and reporting adverse responses.

Regular Training: Improve medical personnel's awareness of adverse reactions and train them regularly to recognize those with ease.

CHAPTER 10: PATIENT EDUCATION

10. 1 Providing Instructions and Rationale

1. Clear Communication:

- Use Clear Language: Make it easy for people to understand by using clear and simple language when giving instructions.

- Avoid Jargon: Ensure that the information is understandable for the patient and minimize the use of medical jargon.

2. Confirm Understanding:

- Ask for Feedback: Seek to promote clarification by motivating patients to ask questions or give their opinion in a bid to confirm understanding of prescribed remedies.

- Repeat Information: Restate important details and request that the patient recap the directions.

3. Written Materials:

- Provide Written Instructions: Provide information in writing, for example, pamphlets and handbooks, to support verbal guidelines.

- Visual Aids: For complicated instructions always use diagrams or visual aids to improve comprehension.

4. Demonstration:

- Show and Tell: Whenever it is feasible, show procedures and/or techniques.

- Patient Participation: /Build confidence by encouraging patients to practice or repeat the actions demonstrated to them.

5. Rationale Explanation:

- Explain the Why: Describe the reason for the particular line of treatment by justifying each instruction.

- Benefits and Risks: What are the advantages when you follow instructions and what problems will arise with failure to follow instructions?

6. Individualized Instructions:

- Tailor to Patient Needs: tailor directions to take into account the patient's health literacy, cand, and culture, preferences.

- Consider Health Literacy: Do not assume that you know what is necessary to explain to them and use simple words.

7. Relevance to Goals:

- Link to Patient Goals: Ensure that the connect instructions lead to the patient's general healthcare aims and wellness.

- Empowerment: Highlight that obedience promotes the patient's empowerment and active participation in the treatment process.

8. Two-Way Communication:

- Encourage Questions: Make sure that patients feel free to ask questions.

- Listen Actively: Practice active listening to ensure you understand the patient's concerns/uncertainties.

9. Encourage Compliance:

- Highlight Importance: The need for adhering to instructions for improved health outcomes.

- Address Barriers: Point out any obstacles that might hinder compliance—such as cost or availability of services.

10. Repeat and Reinforce:

- Repetition: Clarify key messages by repeating them in subsequent interventions.

- Check for Retention: Evaluate if patients remember what they have been taught in between consultations.

11. Multidisciplinary Collaboration:

- Team Communication: Work closely with other healthcare providers in your team to provide an aligned treatment plan on all aspects of your case.

- Consistent Messaging: Check if care plans are consistent with the guidelines given.

12. Cultural Sensitivity:

- Cultural Competence: When giving instruction ensure that you are culturally sensitive by taking into account the patient's culture and beliefs.

- Language Preferences: Respect patients' linguistic choices and offer directions in a suitable language of choice.

13. Follow-Up Plan:

- Establish Follow-Up: Make sure you also clearly outline any need for further appointments, follow-up, or monitoring.

- Contact Information: Give your contact details in case of any complaints arising after the appointment.

14. Documentation:

- Charting Details: Ensure that you document the instructions offered (with or without a rationale) on a medical sheet of a particular patient.

- Communication Notes: Include communication notes on instructions discussions and patient understanding.

10.2 Responding to Patients' concerns/questions.

1. Active Listening:

- Attentive Listening: Direct all your attention to the patient and show him/her that you genuinely understand him.

- Non-Verbal Cues: For instance, you should use nonverbal gestures like nodding to show that you are paying attention or interested in what they have to say.

2. Encourage Open Communication:

- Open-Ended Questions: Utilize open-ended questions to encourage patients to share their concerns/questions

- Non-Judgmental Tone:

3. Clarification:

- Repeat Back: Ensure accurate understanding of the concern by restating it in your own words.

4. Validate Emotions:

- Acknowledge Emotions: Validate the emotions of patients and their concerns as every experience for a patient is different.

- Empathy: Show compassion by articulating any apprehension or uncertainty the patient could be going through.

5. Provide Information:

- Clear and Concise Answers: Ensure that your answers are brief and direct towards particular queries.

- Use Layman's Terms: Use simple language, explain terms in layman's language for easy comprehension, and avoid medical jargon.

6. Rationale Explanation:

- Explain Why: Give reasons why you are giving the patient the information or instructions to enable him/her to understand the rationale for your recommendations.

- Benefits and Risks: Explore possible advantages and disadvantages of various scenarios.

7. Involve the Patient in Decision-Making:
- Shared Decision-Making: Include the patient in decision-making where appropriate, based on their values and desires.
- Discuss Options: Offer various alternatives, and allow the patient to select what suits them best.

8. Collaborate with the Care Team:
- Consult Colleagues: To obtain extra data and ideas one can ask their colleagues and others who may be interested in giving an opinion on the situation at hand.
- Team Approach: Highlight a team-based perspective that includes others in health care settings with appropriate needs.

9. Provide Additional Resources:
- Written Materials: Supplement verbal materials with written texts or credible web sources.

- Support Groups: Refer individuals facing certain health conditions to support groups or counselors.

10. Follow-Up Plan:

- Outline Next Steps: Ensure you specifically describe subsequent processes such as further tests, appointments, and monitoring.

- Contact Information: Give a clear telephone number and email address in case of related queries.

11. Document Interactions:

- Charting Details: Document any concern; question addressed or information added to your patient's medical records.

- Communication Notes: Capture notes on all major discussions discussed and resolved.

12. Timely Follow-Up:

- Scheduled Follow-Up: Arrange for additional visits or telephonic contact for lasting complaints.

- Prompt Responses: Reply fast to patients' calls and questions in due course.

13. Cultural Sensitivity:

- Cultural Competence: Always remember that every culture is different, so use appropriate and culturally sensitive language in your conversations.

- Language Preferences: Respect the languages and offer interpretations if necessary.

CHAPTER 11: LEGAL AND ETHICAL CONSIDERATIONS

11.1 Scope of Practice

1. Definition:

- Professional Boundaries: Practice scope outlines health care professionals' limits of practice within whom they can administer services based on educational attainments and qualifications.

2. Education and Training:

Qualifications:

It depends on a healthcare professional's education, qualifications, and training.

- Continuing Education: Ongoing learning and development can further extend their expertise.

3. Legal and Regulatory Framework:

- Licensing Boards: The regulatory bodies and licensing boards determine and enforce the scope of practices for health care professions.

- Legal Standards: This involves legal compliance and defines the scope.

4. Specialty Areas:

- Specialized Practice: Certain healthcare professionals work in unique fields, narrowing down their general occupation.

- Certifications: The scope could also be narrower in specialized areas depending on the relevant certificates.

5. Clinical Procedures:

- Authorized Interventions: The scope describes clinical procedures and interventions an expert is permitted to exercise.

- Limitations: Well circumscribed to assure safety and quality of service.

6. Prescription Authority:
- Medication Prescribing: If professionals can prescribe drugs or not.

- Drug Classes: This is because some can impose constraintsregardingo drugs they are allowed to prescribe.

7. Assessment and Diagnosis:
- Diagnostic Procedures: Provides an overview of how far professionals can go in carrying out diagnostic assessments.

- Limitations on Diagnosis: Some of these professions are also able to make a diagnosis in their specialization, whereas some of them have to work together with other healthcare providers.

8. Collaboration and Referral:
- Interprofessional Collaboration: Promotes interprofessional collaborative practice for total patient care.

- Referral Processes: Specifies referral process of patients to specialists when necessary.

9. Ethical Standards:
- Ethical Guidelines: Health care providers operate ethically within scope.
- Confidentiality: Sets out confidentiality issues relating to information about patients.

10. Patient Education:
- Health Promotion:This may entail tasks involving health promotion and preventive patient education.
- Informed Consent: Before gaining informed consent, professionals see that patients understand what interventions are under their care.

11. Scope Expansion:
- Legislative Changes: However, the cope could change with legislative adjustments that may allow wider responsibilities.

- Advanced Practice Roles: Autonomy may be included in the extended scope for advanced practice roles.

12. Continuing Competence: Professional development emphasizes the need for continuous improvement to sustain competency and some professions may also require recertification or recredentialisation to show that they have maintained competence to remain valid.

13. Quality Improvement: DEDICATION: Incorporates encouraging participation in quality improvement undertakings to raise healthcare for patients.

AUDIT AND FEEDBACK: It might entail periodical audit and feedback measures focusing on the observance of standards.

14. Adherence to Guidelines: Evidence-based clinical guidelines relevant to professionals' scopes

(Clinical Guidelines) and National standards (National Standards) facilitate consistency in care delivery.

15. Cultural Competence: It boosts cultural competency, including a variety of patients' cultural backgrounds and adapting the care as necessary.

16. Interdisciplinary Collaboration: Team-based care is a model of practice where the health workers team up to deliver comprehensive and integrated patient-centered care.

11. 2 Informed Consent in Healthcare

1. Definition:

- Voluntary Agreement: Informed consent is an informed and autonomous decision of a competent patient to submit himself or herself to a particular therapy or medical procedure based on the disclosure of necessary data.

2. Components of Informed Consent:

- Nature of the Procedure: Therefore, briefly describe the essence, goals, and characteristics of the planned procedure or therapy.

- Risks and Benefits: State possible risks, benefits, and alternatives of the intervention.

- Alternative Options: Discuss other treatment options or interventions one can seek.

- Questions and Clarifications: Allow the people concerned to inquire about the proposed intervention.

3. Competence and Capacity:

- Assessment: Ensure that the person is mentally alert and able to comprehend the data presented.

- Assistance if Needed: Where possible, engage with family members and guardians for further clarification about the information under consideration.

4. Voluntariness:

- Freedom of Choice: Make it clear that providing consent is a free will act with no pressurizing or coercing of any party involved.

- Withdrawal of Consent: Inform people they can withdraw consent anytime and no penalty will be applied.

5. Timing of Consent:

- Advance Consent: Get informed consent before any intervention when feasible.

- Emergency Situations: Ensure information is given and consent is sought as soon as possible in case of emergencies.

6. Documentation:

- Written Consent Form: Obtain a written consent form that clearly explains the main aspects of the surgery, potential effects, and advantages as well as alternative options.

- Signatures: Use the consent form signature as proof of consent.

- Witness Signatures: Provide witness signature(s) if necessary to authenticate the informed consent process.

7. Communication:

- Clear Communication: Avoid using medicinal jargon to enhance understanding and simplify communication.

- Interactive Discussion: Promote a discussion involving an interaction wherein the person is in a position to raise worries and queries.

8. Cultural Sensitivity:

- Cultural Competence: Ensure you are sensitive to their culture, look at how these individuals react to things.

- Language Considerations: Ensure the individual's preferred language is communicated with, and include interpretation services where possible.

9. Pediatric Consent:

- Parental or Guardian Consent: Obtain informed consent (for minors) from parents and/or legal guardians.

- Assent: As much as possible, get the child's consent or agreement depending on his/her age and maturity, when necessary.

10. Special Populations:

- Vulnerable Populations: Give special care and sensitivity while seeking these vulnerable population's assent like the aging or weak.

11. Continuous Communication:

- Ongoing Updates: Inform people of any adjustments made regarding the treatment and other new details that could change their minds.

- Reassurance: Build trust, reassure, and provide support during informed consent.

12. Documentation Completeness:

- Record Keeping: Ensure the informed consent process is well documented in the individual's medical record.

- Date and Time: Put also the date and time of the consent discussion and signature.

13. Adherence to Ethical Principles:

- Autonomy: Promote individual self-determination and grant people the right to determine what healthcare options they need without interference from others.

- Beneficence and Non-Maleficence: In addition, the proposed intervention must be made in the patient's interests and never cause any harm.

14. Periodic Review:

- Review Consent: Informed consent should be periodically reviewed and updated in case of any changes in the treatment plan or new interventions proposed.

15. Educational Materials:

- Supplementary Information: Supply additional learning resources like books, pamphlets, or films for comprehension purposes.

CHAPTER 12: CONTINUOUS EDUCATION AND TRAINING

12. Continuous education and training in healthcare.

1. Lifelong Learning Culture:

- Promote Continuous Learning: Create a learning culture in healthcare organizations where continued education becomes a life-long process of commitment.

- Professional Growth: Reinforce the point that life-long learning impacts career development and the provision of quality services for patients.

2. Continuing Professional Development (CPD):
- Structured Programs: Develop well-defined CPD programs based on current practices to keep up with the changing demands of healthcare workers.
- Multi-Modal Approaches: Use different modalities such as workshops, seminars, online courses, and conferences to cater to learners with varying preferences.

3. Individualized Learning Plans:
- Assessment of Needs: Regular assessments may be done to discover specific learning needs or tastes of an individual.
- Tailored Plans: Create an individualized plan for each professional development goal.

4. Technology Integration:
- E-Learning Platforms: Harness the use of e-learning platforms and digital resources for flexible, accessible, and self-paced learning.

- Virtual Simulations: Use technology such as virtual simulations to provide realistic practical experiences.

5. Certification and Credentialing:
- Encourage Certification: Provide incentives for healthcare professionals to obtain appropriate certifications in their areas of specialization.
- Recognition: Recognise and congratulate individuals who have achieved certifications or advanced degrees to continue motivating learning.

6. Interprofessional Collaboration:
- Collaborative Learning: Encourage interprofessional collaboration during training sessions to share information and views.
- Team-Based Training: Organise team-based training for improved communications and improved teamwork among health care providers.

7. Mentorship Programs:

- Experienced Mentors: Develop a network of mentoring where senior experts would share their experience with beginners in terms of professional growth.

- Knowledge Transfer: Mentor other teachers, promote knowledge sharing between teachers, and share a teacher's practical insight with others.

8. Regular Workshops and Seminars:

- Topic-Relevant Sessions: Hold frequent sessions for discussing recent changes in healthcare matters, trending technologies, as well as scientifically established tactics.

- Guest Speakers: Organize conferences for inviting guest speakers, specialists, and thought leaders to share ideas and experiences with the health community.

9. Research Engagement:

- Encourage Research Participation: Involve healthcare providers in research projects so that they can assist and enhance their specific areas of expertise.

- Research Literacy: Train health professionals in research literacy such that they review and utilize research-based information.

10. Regulatory Updates:

- Stay Informed on Regulations: Keep healthcare providers updated on new developments in regulations, standards of practice, and guidelines.

- Compliance Training: Carry out regular compliance training to confirm adherence to the code of ethics and laws.

11. Feedback Mechanisms:

- Evaluation and Feedback: Put in place processes for post-training program assessment and feedback collection from trainees.

- Continuous Improvement: Constantly use feedback to fine-tune the design and provision of instruction.

12. Recognition and Incentives:

- Acknowledgement: Appreciate and recognize the healthcare practitioners who undertake continuing education.

- Incentive Programs: Think about a reward policy in the form of a prize or professional development grant, which may motivate learners continuously.

13. Flexibility and Accessibility:

- Flexible Learning Opportunities: Offer flexible learning chances with a view that healthcare workers have different timetables and commitments.

- Online Resources: Remote or busy professionals can have access to education resources through online platforms.

14. Leadership Support:
- Leadership Advocacy: Push towards constant training at various points of management stressing the significance of qualified and well-trained healthcare team members.
- Resource Allocation: Provide funding and support for continuing education programs.

15. Regular Assessments:
- Competency Assessments: Engage in regular competency assessments to discover shortcomings that should be addressed through enhanced training.
- Feedback for Improvement: Tailoring education and training program according to assessment results.

12. 2 Incident report and analysis in healthcare facilities.

1. Definition:

- Incident Reporting: The formal recording and evaluation of adverse events, mistakes, and close calls in a healthcare facility.

2. Importance of Incident Reporting:

- Continuous Improvement: One of the main means for continuous advancement in ensuring patient safety and quality of care.

- Identifying Trends: Identify patterns and trends among incidents that can be addressed in advance.

3. Reporting Culture:

- Encourage Open Reporting: Establish a safe reporting environment wherein healthcare providers can report incidents without being condemned or punished.

- Anonymous Reporting: Ensure anonymity in whistleblowing processes to foster authenticity and openness.

4. Types of Incidents:
- Adverse Events: Disclose adverse events or injuries suffered by patients.
- Near Misses: Report incidents which did not lead to harm, but posed risks of occurring.
- Errors: This includes such errors as those associated with medication, documentation, and procedure.

5. Incident Reporting System:
- Establish a System: Create a simple incident report management tool for the use of all hospital staff.
- Electronic Reporting: Use electronic reporting systems to simplify the process, and improve the accuracy of data collection.

6. Reporting Responsibilities:

- All Staff Involvement: It should be clearly stated that all healthcare workers need to have an assigned role for reporting incidents, ranging from the first responders to administration.

- Timeframe: Set up deadlines for informing incidents to ensure proper documentation.

7. Initial Incident Report:

- Immediate Documentation: Ensure that basic information about an incident is documented directly by indicating the day, time, place, and parties involved without awaiting any detailed report.

- Objective Language: Provide detailed, objective, and factual accounts of the incident, and avoid terms such as 'blame' and 'judgment'.

8. Investigation Team:

- Multidisciplinary Team: Convene a multi-discipline committee to inquire on the reported cases.

- Diversity of Perspectives: Have individuals with varied opinions carry out in-depth analysis.

9. Root Cause Analysis (RCA):
- Systematic Approach: Engage in systematic RCA in identifying the causes of occurrences.
- Contributing Factors: Investigate underlying causes like human, organizational, and environmental matters.

10. Corrective and Preventive Actions:
- Action Planning: Conduct a root cause analysis and develop corrective and preventive action plans.
- Implementation: Take corrective action immediately upon identifying problems.

11. Communication:
- Transparent Communication: Issue detailed communication about incident findings and actions taken transparently to all concerned parties.

- Learn from Incidents: Put the accent on incident reports as an occasion for organizational learning and development.

12. Continuous Monitoring:
- Ongoing Surveillance: Establish a continuous monitoring mechanism to ensure that corrective actions are effective.
- Feedback Loops: Set up communication lines for informing employees about the advancements in incident mitigation and improvements.

13. Feedback to Reporters:
- Acknowledgment: Assure persons reporting incidents that they are being appreciated by praising them.
- Anonymity Maintenance: Provide feedback to reporters only if that is necessary and in case it involves keeping their identities anonymous.

14. Legal and Ethical Considerations:

- Legal Obligations: Ensure adherence to legal duties involving accident reports and observe regulatory regulations.

- Ethical Obligations: Ensure ethical values during reporting and maintain confidentiality of patient data.

15. Education and Training:

- Training Programs: Continuous education and training of healthcare personnel on the procedures of incident reporting and the need for lessons learned.

- Simulation Training: Use incident scenarios in simulations as part of the staff preparedness process.

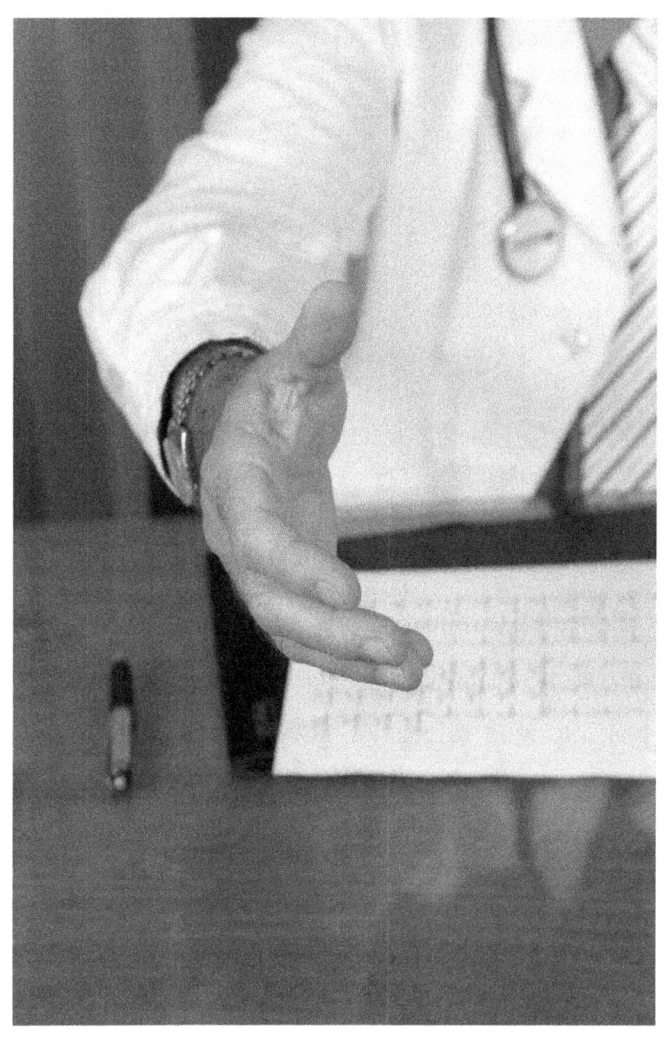

CHAPTER 13: EMERGENCIES AND COMPLICATIONS

13.1 Identifying and managing adverse reactions in healthcare.

1. Early Recognition:

- Educate Healthcare Providers: Educate healthcare providers on how to detect early warning signs of possible side effects or adverse reactions as they occur, or shortly after medical or surgical intervention.

- Vigilance: Promote alertness regarding changes in the body reaction of each patient to the medication.

2. Common Adverse Reactions:
- Identification: List common side effects from particular medications/ interventions.

- Severity Grading: t a severity criteria for assessment of adverse reactions to formulate necessary interventions.

3. Vigilant Monitoring:
- Continuous Monitoring: Highlight ongoing surveillance, particularly during critical processes such as surgeries and administering drugs with noted adverse consequences.
- Vital Signs: Frequently check for significant variations in vital signs suggestive of serious side effects. management using computer applications has made decision-making easier and enhanced performance.

4. Emergency Response Training:
- Simulation Training: Simulation training can be conducted on health care providers on how these emergencies from adverse drug reactions are managed.

- Team Coordination: Ensure effective teamwork among members, especially during emergency response situations.

5. Rapid Intervention Protocols:
- Establish Protocols: The need for the development of rapid intervention protocols aimed at guiding healthcare providers on how to respond to adverse reactions must be realized.
- Clear Communication: Provide open lines of communication leading to activation of the emergency response team in case necessary.

6. Documentation of Adverse Events:
- Accurate Documentation: Reinforce the need for proper and prompt recording of such occurrences entailing information about the kind of reaction, steps taken, and effect on the individual.
- Report to Authorities: Report all serious adverse events to appropriate health authorities according to applicable laws.

7. Risk-Benefit Assessment:

- Continuous Risk-Benefit Evaluation: Motivate health care providers to conduct continuous risk-utility analysis of interventions as compared with undesirable responses.

- Informed Decision-Making: Include patients in an educated treatment choice discussion and discuss some expected side effects.

8. Anticipation of Potential Complications:

- Preventive Measures: Pre-administration of drugs to prevent side effects could be regarded as a measure of prevention in light of expected adverse reactions.

- Patient Education: Inform patients of the possible risks and also tell them what symptoms they should report after the treatment.

9. Allergy Assessment:

- Prior Allergy History: Record patients' prior history of allergies in detail, to prevent allergic reactions among vulnerable patients.

- Allergy Testing: In case of need, consider allergy testing to confirm some allergies specifically.

10. Adverse Reaction Response Teams:
- Multidisciplinary Teams: Create cross-discipline adverse reaction response committees with professionals from various fields.
- Timely Consultations: Ensure efficient and prompt meetings with specialists in the management of severe side effects.

11. Post-Event Debriefing:
- Debriefing Sessions: Carry out post-event debriefings of managing adverse reactions, areas for improvement, and psychosocial counseling of health providers.
- Continuous Learning: Incorporate debriefing sessions into the adverse event management process as avenues of continual learning and development.

12. Patient Follow-Up:

- Post-Reaction Monitoring: Establish post-reaction monitoring measures to monitor patient conditions for delayed or repeated effects.

- Long-Term Follow-Up: Develop long-term follow-up programs for patients reporting severe AEs.

13. Quality Improvement Initiatives:

- Root Cause Analysis: Do root cause analysis of severe adverse events to uncover systematic problems and avert the repetitive nature of these conditions."

- Quality Improvement Plans: Conduct root cause analysis leading to the development and implementation of quality management strategies which will be used in improving the situation.

14. Communication with Patients:

- Open Communication: Ensure that you communicate openly and frankly with your patients and their families about any adverse reactions encountered and explain why they occur.

- Follow-Up Care Plans: Work together with patients in developing follow-up care plans for managing adverse effects that may persist after discharge.

15. Regulatory Compliance:

- Adherence to Regulations: Require healthcare providers to follow regulatory guidelines on adverse reactions reporting and management."

- Documentation Standards: Ensure that requirements for documenting adverse reaction incidents for compliance and accountability purposes are adhered to with emphasis.

13. 2 Healthcare Emergency Response Protocols

1. Emergency Preparedness Planning:

- Comprehensive Plans: Prepare broad-based emergency response measures for different kinds of emergencies such as cardiac arrest, respiratory distress, and trauma.

- Regular Updates: Update the emergency response protocol periodically to meet the latest standards.

2. Emergency Response Team Activation:

- Clear Activation Criteria: Establish specific metrics that will trigger the deployment of emergency teams as well as indicate the need for immediate action.

- Communication Procedures: Put in place reliable communication mechanisms that will swiftly call for the activation of the right respondents team.

3. Role Assignments:
- Clear Roles and Responsibilities: Assign distinct duties to every individual in the emergency response team.
- Training on Roles: Make sure that each team member is trained on their role as well as emergency duties assigned.

4. Rapid Assessment and Triage:
- Immediate Assessment: Train health professionals to conduct quick assessments for patients in an emergency state and allocate remedies according to urgency.
- Triage Protocols: Use triage protocols to rank patients and distribute resources accordingly.

5. Basic Life Support (BLS):
- Early BLS Interventions: Highlight BLS interventions like CPR, and defibrillation, which emphasize early start up.
- Training Certification: Healthcare professionals, should always have their BLS updated.

6. Advanced Life Support (ALS):
- Prompt ALS Activation: Call ALS quickly when necessary.
- Skill Proficiency: Periodically reevaluate and update skills of health care providers in ALS treatment including intubation and medication provision.

7. Communication Systems:
- Reliable Communication Channels: Put in place trustworthy channels of communication that enable seamless collaboration among team players and agree on some emergency codes.
- Emergency Alerts: Ensure that the health facility has alert dissemination systems.

8. Emergency Equipment Readiness:
- Equipment Checks: Carry out frequent inventories focusing on the functionality of emergency equipment such as defibrillators, airway handling apparatus, and medications.

- Maintenance Protocols: Introduce a maintenance protocol on emergency equipment, to be solved in good time.

9. Evacuation Plans:
- Evacuation Routes: In case of emergencies that warrant relocating of patients as well as staff, develop and communicate clear evacuation routes.
- Training Exercises: Organically hold regular drills for evacuation of medical personnel so that they can be aware of procedures to be undertaken as emergencies.

10. Debriefing and Continuous Improvement:
- Post-Emergency Debriefing: Conduct debriefing sessions every time there is an emergency to analyze what was done, identify gaps that need filling, and also offer emotional support to the team.
- Quality Improvement Initiatives: Improve the current protocols for emergency response by using data from debriefing sessions.

11. Interdisciplinary Collaboration:

- Team Collaboration: Encourage interdisciplinary collaboration in emergencies through enhanced communication and coordination by different types of health workers.

- Training Scenarios: Consider interdisciplinary training scenarios for scenario-based simulations aimed at teamwork.

12. External Resource Coordination:

- Liaison with External Services: Develop ways of collaborating with offsite emergency service providers like ambulance services and community emergency response agencies.

- Information Exchange: Ensure seamless communication of health information among in-house teams and external services.

13. Family and Patient Communication:

- Clear Communication with Families: Devise communications plan about emergencies for updating families on patients' condition and ensuring their concerns.

- Designated Liaisons: Designate specific contacts to interface with families and address their concerns.

14. Documentation Standards:
- Thorough Documentation: Stress the necessity of full documentation of all response's actions.
- Post-Event Reporting: Create a process that calls for reporting and evaluation of emergencies and identifies areas for improvement.

15. Regulatory Compliance:
- Adherence to Regulations: Make sure these protocols are locally, regionally, and nationally lawful.
- Regular Audits: Perform routine audits to determine whether emergency management procedures are being adhered to or not and fill any loopholes.

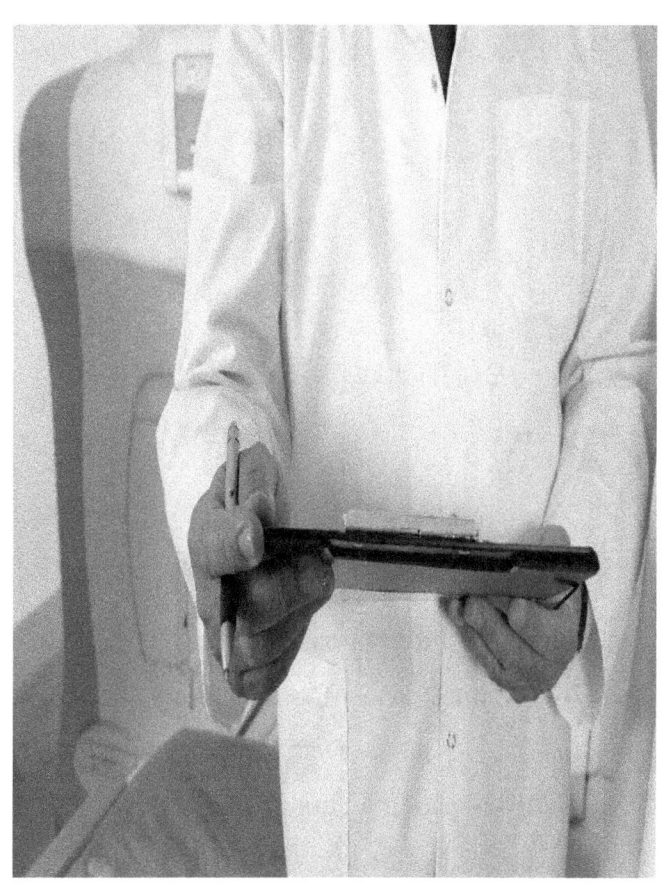

CHAPTER 14: FUTURE TRENDS IN INJECTION ADMINISTRATION

14. 1 Technological Advancement in Healthcare

1. Electronic Health Records (EHRs):

- Comprehensive Patient Data: Through EHRs, comprehensive information about a patient is stored digitally creating ease of accessibility as well as coordination of the same for improved quality of services to that patient in question.

- Interoperability: The improvements seek to make cross-referencing possible so that the patient can share information with other health facilities easily.

2. Telemedicine and Telehealth:

- Virtual Consultations: Providing telemedicine ensures that a patient can obtain consultation with a healthcare provider remotely thereby increasing medical accessibility.

- Remote Monitoring: Improvements in telehealth can assist in monitoring the vital signs and some other aspects of a patient's health.

3. Robotics in Surgery:
- Minimally Invasive Procedures: With the help of robotic-assisted surgery, patients can undertake minimally invasive and more precision surgeries which in turn reduce post-operational recovery time.

- Surgeon Assistance: During these complicated surgeries, robots can assist surgeons with improved visualization and better control.

4. Wearable Health Devices:
- Continuous Monitoring: Wearable devices like fitness trackers or smart watches constantly measure health-related indicators e.g. heart rate, activities, and sleep.

- Patient Engagement: Through wearables, patients increase their motivation and get instant results to support healthy lifestyles.

5. 3D Printing in Medicine:

- Customized Implants: There is also customization of prosthetics, implants, and anatomic models for planning surgery using this technology (i.e., 3D printing).

- Tissue Engineering: The improved 3D printing facilitates bioprinting used to construct living tissue and organs.

6. Personalized Medicine:

- Genomic Analysis: Through personalized medicine, patients' treatment plans are tailored specifically for them relying on their unique gene profile.

- Targeted Therapies: The recent advancement in molecular profiling enables the selection of patient-specific molecular targets for superior and personalized therapy.

7. Augmented and Virtual Reality (AR/VR):

- Medical Training: Medical training has been improved through the adoption of augmented reality and virtual reality technologies making simulated procedures and surgeries more intense.

- Patient Education: Patient instruction can be improved by providing a virtual reality experience for them to understand what is wrong with their body and how it can be treated.

8. Internet of Things (IoT):

- Connected Devices: IoT enables connection between medical equipment and allows for their real-time remote monitoring and sharing of information.

- Smart Hospitals: Smart hospitals become possible as a result of connected IoT applications which improve efficiencies.

9. Nanomedicine:
- Precision Drug Delivery: Precise and effective medication administration is possible with nanotechnology in medicine.
- Diagnostic Nanosensors: Diagnostics have been enhanced by nanoscale sensors for early disease diagnosis.

10. Blockchain in Healthcare:
- Data Security: In healthcare, blockchain helps ensure data security and integrity through using a distributed and untamperable ecosystem.
- Interoperability: Interoperability can be achieved through blockchain that provides an interchangeable, standardized, and safe channel for sharing healthcare information.

11. Health Information Exchange (HIE):
- Inter-Organizational Data Sharing: Healthcare Information Exchanges (HIEs) foster safe transfer of patient data across different medical facilities.

- Coordinated Care: The improved technical evolution of HIE leads to enhanced coordination among the professionals and patient-centricity.

12. Mobile Health (mHealth):
- Health Apps: There are mobile health apps that support health status monitoring, medication adherence, and wellbeing.
- Remote Accessibility: The mHealth technologies assist in supporting the remote provision of care services, leading to enhanced patient engagement and empowerment for self-management.

13. Genomic Editing:
- CRISPR Technology: CRISPR gene editing has enabled doctors to modify exact genes to treat different types of genetic diseases.
- Gene Therapy: New advances in genomic editing have made it possible to develop gene therapies for many different forms of illnesses.

14. Continuous Research and Development:

- Emerging Technologies: This means that there is always newer technology in the health sector, calling for continuous research and advancements.

- Integration into Clinical Practice: Patient care continues to improve through continuous monitoring and incorporation of newly developed technology for the clinic.

14.2 Evolving Standards And Best Practices.

1. Patient-Centered Care:

- Individualized Treatment Plans: Best practices are founded on patient–centered approaches where each patient deserves a unique plan based on their personal preferences, values, and circumstances.

- Shared Decision-Making: Stimulate joint decision-making of healthcare service givers and clients, thus creating an open and cooperative care environment.

2. Interdisciplinary Collaboration:

- Team-Based Approach: Interdisciplinary working helps enhance communication between different health care service providers.

- Care Coordination: Evolving standards concern enhancing the quality of care and care coordination across specialties in a comprehensive management of the patient.

3. Evidence-Based Practice:

- Informed Decision-Making: Focus on emphasizing the application of recent evidence in decision-making to ensure that healthcare practices have scientific ground. #

- Regular Updates: Evolving standards refer to a process whereby clinical guidelines are constantly reviewed and updated using current evidence and scientific information.

4. Continuous Quality Improvement:

- Quality Metrics: Continuously introduce quality enhancement strategies that are based on measurable outcomes used in monitoring healthcare service delivery.

- Feedback Loops: Enhanced standards allow for closed-loop systems whereby providers may learn through results, subsequently improving their practice.

5. Patient Safety Initiatives:

- Culture of Safety: Creating a culture of safety in healthcare organizations that allows for reporting and analysis of incidents can improve patient safety.

- Adherence to Protocols: Emerging standards address various aspects of compliance with safety procedures, reducing mistakes and vulnerabilities.

6. Health Information Security:

- Data Protection: Ensure that health information is well protected. Update information according to modern data protection and privacy standards.

- Cybersecurity Protocols: Be aware of emerging cybersecurity regulations to protect data and private medical information.

7. Cultural Competence:

- Culturally Sensitive Care: When delivering competent standards of care cultural congruence should be observed in recognition that patients may come from different cultures and belief systems.

- Training Programs: Healthcare professionals' cultural competence and sensitivity are ensured by evolving standards where there are continuous training programs.

8. Telehealth Integration:
- Accessible Healthcare: Telehealth should be regarded as a natural aspect of the health system with its purpose of making health services more accessible while increasing the comfort of patient care.
- Regulatory Compliance: Developing guidelines include the revision of rules to guarantee that the use of telemedicine in traditional healthcare practice is secure and successful.

9. Ethical Decision-Making:

- Ethical Guidelines: Ethical standards are at the center of any best practice whereby health care practitioners make informed choices concerning patients' interests and rights.

- Ethics Committees: Changing standards advocate for ethics committees to address complex ethical issues and offer guides in difficult conditions.

10. Patient Engagement Strategies:

- Health Literacy: Develop measures for improving the health literacy of patients and facilitate active involvement of patients in decisions concerning their care.

- Digital Health Tools: Moving standards drive the use of digital health apps for patient engagement in managing health and well-being.

11. Advanced Care Planning:

- Early Discussions: Such practices involve discussion with patients early on about advance care planning, documenting their preferred end-of-life care options, and honoring them.

- Regular Reevaluation: Improved standards emphasize periodic scrutiny of advanced care plans for updated preferences of patients over time.

12. Standardized Communication Protocols:
- Effective Communication: Develop standardized communication processes among health teams to eliminate errors in data sharing.
- Interoperability Initiatives: Emerging standards are geared towards increasing the level of healthcare interoperability to enable smooth communication across disparate healthcare information systems.

13. Professional Development:
- Continuous Training: Continuous professional development should be encouraged in health care; hence professionals must remain updated with recent research, technology, and best practices.

- Credentialing Requirements: In this regard, evolving standards could involve changing credentialing requirements to take into account developments in medical knowledge and technology.

14. Value-Based Care:
- Outcome-Based Metrics: Movement toward more patient-centered care models with attention to quality and outcomes instead of the quantity of healthcare services offered.
- Payment Reforms: Standards are evolving, discussing payment reforms that provide aligned incentives for the delivery of high-quality and affordable services.

Conclusion

In summary, safe injection requires a systematic and patient-oriented approach that encompasses various components to assure the safety of the patient and the efficacy of the medication. Key considerations include:

1. Foundational Knowledge: As a prelude to this, it is essential to gain basic knowledge of anatomy, equipment, and techniques. Aspects such as assessment of veins or muscles, selection of adequate needles and syringes, and maintenance of sterile technique play a significant role.

2. Patient Preparation: Such things as preparing the patient both physically and emotionally explaining the procedure and getting informed consent are a lot to a positive and safe injection experience for the patient.

3. Technical Proficiency: Insertion techniques, needle depth and angles along with specialized ones like Z-Track minimize such complications and leakages.

4. Safety Protocols: Above all, safety regulations such as hand hygiene and safe disposal of sharps should be observed. Monitoring complications continuously allows for timely remediation should problems arise.

5. Communication and Documentation: Good practices involve clear communication with patients, accurately charting administrative details, and reporting adverse reactions promptly which ensure comprehensive and safe health care.

6. Emergency Preparedness: Healthcare providers need to be prepared in advance for unexpected situations since they directly affect the safety of patients.

7. Utilization of Technology: The use of modern technologies including electronic health records and telemedicine improves accuracy, convenience, and overall quality of service delivery.

8. Ethical Considerations: The above are essential principles that aid in creating a professional yet patient-orientated approach.

9. Continuous Improvement: Continuous quality improvements, staying abreast with the best practices, and complying with changing standards ensure the provision of quality, safe care.